# HEART TO HEART RESUSCITATION

## A MEMOIR

**Victor Montgomery, III, MAEd, M-RAS, CMAC**

For information, contact

MSI Press, LLC

1760-F Airline Hwy #203

Hollister, CA 95023

Copyeditor: Betty Lou Leaver

Cover design & layout: Opeyemi Ikuborije

LCCN: 2023916812

ISBN: 9781957354354

# CONTENTS

# Acknowledgements

All my love and appreciation and a huge thank you go to my wife and steadfast partner, Diane Joy Montgomery, for all the hours enthusiastically sustaining me and praying for this book to be published to feed hope and encouragement to our nation's veterans, their families, and friends.

To my good friends, staff and co-workers in counseling centers around the country, friends at the VA Medical Center in Canandaigua, New York (Michele Rice, Bob Iredale, Karrah Bruder, and Amy Foster), California clinic teams (Liz Hagaman, Lauren, Lynn & Larry Vaughan, Neil Sommer and Marianne Abalone) for all the years of camaraderie and working together each day with a positive treatment team spirit and vision, thank you!

To my friends, confidants, and ministers: Tom Sommers, Russ & Carol Milnes, Rev. Powell Lemons, Chaplain Glen Davis, the late Rev. Eric & Gladys Johnson and Rev. Dr. Al Vom Steeg, my brothers and sisters in Christian ministry. To my VA Medical Center colleagues on the Crisis Hotlines (Bill Cerveny, Terry Taylor and the late Roger Cheney) for their support and engaging enthusiasm for me to publish my books. And, in memory of my good friend George Mead, who died tragically in a motorcycle accident in 2017. His son committed suicide after three tours in Iraq and Afghanistan.

And finally, a special thanks to Dr. Betty Lou Leaver, Managing Editor of MSI Press, LLC, for her belief in me and in the cause of spreading hope and encouragement to our nation's veterans and for editorial assistance in writing and publishing about the hearts, minds, and souls of our great American warriors and their families.

# Author's Note

Even the toughest of the tough, the "true grit" combat warrior decorated for valor can over time succumb to lying on a field hospital cot in the fetal position with nothing left to give. Wherever a war is fought, be it in the sandy arid deserts, jungles, and mangrove swamps of Vietnam, the mountains, forests, and woodlands of Korea, or the amphibious landings on the islands of the Pacific, the enormity of the human cruelty and tragic events seen and experienced can exceed many veterans' abilities to cope. Over the years, fire fights, mortar attacks, roadside explosives, and sniper fire in Iraq and Afghanistan eventually take their toll. So do multiple deployments, sleepless nights, witnessing of unrelenting carnage, and the loss of buddies. Many warriors share nothing, say nothing.

Today, tens of thousands suffer in silence. Battle fatigue, shell shock, Post-Traumatic Stress Disorder (PTSD), Traumatic Brain Injury (TBI), depression, anxiety, and alcohol dependence, are silent killers.

These invisible combat veterans take cover in plain sight. They return home from combat zones lost in a deep abyss of confusion, darkness, and desperation. For many, the readjustment to civilian life is often an impossibility without the proper help and motivation.

And so, the struggles begin. As with any war, the battle against addiction destroys families and claims lives—tens of thousands of lives.

*Heart to Heart Resuscitation* (H2HR) is based on my personal experiences in counseling, coaching, mentoring, and ministering to combat veterans for over 20 years. It reflects my observations of the events and conversations in my practice as well as the steps, strategies, and measures taken to bring our military men and women help and hope.

In this book, I honor with anonymity the veterans, families and survivors who have entrusted me with their heartfelt stories. To protect their privacy, I have changed the names of individuals but have altered only identifying characteristics; their stories are true.

# Introduction

The window of opportunity to make a difference to someone whose life may hang in the balance can literally be a matter of seconds. Through this book, I hope to share the unique, tested method of crisis intervention that I refer to as "Heart to Heart Resuscitation" and use to overcome the combat veterans' immediate, life-threatening darkness of depression and suicidal thoughts. My number one priority is to get veterans to safety. By encouraging, motivating and mentoring suffering veterans, I help them find the strength, self-determination, and support to get help and out of danger. The intention of this book is to share the straightforward, down-to-earth advice infused with encouragement and hope that I offer to my veteran clients.

## For whom did I write this book?

Vietnam veterans, as well as veterans of the more recent wars in Iraq and Afghanistan are today living on city streets, in cars, and in the nation's homeless shelters. Some are so desperate they commit crimes and are going to prison. Many struggling vets or family and friends in the neighborhood end up calling hospital emergency rooms, psychiatric nurses, 911, 211, or the Veterans Administration (VA) hotline (988+1) for help and advice.

An equally large number are reluctant to contact anyone at all. Account after account reports veterans locking themselves in their rooms, not coming out for days at a time. When they do reach out for help to a hotline or emergency department, they explain, "Asking for help is like saying I've failed my mission."

When veterans call a clinic expressing symptoms of depressive illnesses that interfere with their everyday life functioning, they are made aware that professional medical treatment *teams* will be made available. A call for help on behalf of a veteran is highly recommended when the veteran has thoughts of or mentions a plan or intention to harm himself or herself. Even if there is no suicide ideation, the vet may be experiencing a "crisis" of a different nature: unrelenting psychological (mental) and physiological (body) pain, feelings of helplessness and hopelessness, effects of substance abuse or other addictions, feeling out of control, or need for anger management.

Mental health clinicians around the country are seeing significant substance abuse cases, particularly alcohol dependency, among veterans. Some veterans exposed to trauma and negative experiences in war zones are self-medicating with alcohol and other drugs at a high rate. After coming home, these veterans seldom report, at least at the beginning, any mental health problems. Often it is several months and even several years after veterans settle into their lives at home and work that delayed symptoms of anxiety, panic, rage, anger, depression, and insomnia begin to appear or become recurrent in their daily routines. Increasing alcohol intake and the taking of illicit street drugs, such as marijuana, opiates, cocaine, methamphetamines, and pain killers often become daily scourges.

Domestic violence and marital and family disputes are other ways veterans show their pain and depression. Marriages are in jeopardy; jobs are lost or never found; financial difficulties surface; and children begin to fear for their safety in their own homes.

An increasing number of veterans come home from the conflicts in Iraq and Afghanistan already diagnosed with post-traumatic stress disorder or traumatic brain injury (TBI). After months and even years of experiencing tours of nighttime firefights, picking up enemy bodies, finding baby toys and articles of children's clothing on the floors of suspected terrorists' houses, combat veterans, unsurprisingly in rapidly increasing numbers, turn to antidepressants daily to control and ease the effects of lengthy and repeated tours. *Heart to Heart Resuscitation* has important information for these vets, those who work with them, and those who are close to them.

So, who are you? Active duty military? Veteran? Family member? Friend? Co-worker? Registered nurse? Licensed practical nurse? Therapist? Medical doctor? Counselor? Psychologist? Graduate student? Psychiatrist? Combat medic? Addiction therapist? Social worker? Educator? Battle buddy? Emergency medical technician? Fire person? A veteran missing your buddies, no one to have your back? Care givers tired out by veterans who keep relapsing? A neighbor or co-worker of a veteran who needs help? *Heart to Heart Resuscitation* was written for all of you.

## What can you find in this book?

This book attempts to answer difficult questions about why so many veterans are dying by their own hands. The answers are found in understanding the psychological wounds of war, learning some terms that may be unfamiliar, and identifying high-risk signs for suicide, The reader can find plain words with careful description about how to recognize what defines a veteran's need for counseling, what signs to look for, and what to do when you discover them.

In the following chapters you also will find real stories of raw emotion, expressed by men and women veterans, as well as family, friends, and callers pleading for help before it is too late. I will move you through the poignant, uncensored personal stories shared with me by desperate veterans coming into Group Room #2 at the clinic where I work, stories reflecting many combat experiences. Some vets in these stories have already hurt themselves and need immediate emergency rescue while others are confused and cannot find their way in life. And some just want someone to listen.

Most important, I will try to point out the steps and strategies in the veterans' stories that can help them recover. If you are a veteran, I will do my utmost, drawing on my long experience with other veterans, to guide you on a path that will lead you from the darkness and anguish of pain and suffering to growth and resuscitation, using the Montgomery Model of Heart to Heart Resuscitation. That same path can be walked by a loved one together with a veteran. I know our journey together calls for strength and courage, but I also know you have both. You or your loved one is a genuine American hero.

## What is the Montgomery Model of Heart to Heart Resuscitation?

Heart-to-heart resuscitation is about presence. It is about you or someone close to you. My mission as a teacher and therapist, whether I am face-to-face with someone in my clinic or talking on the phone, is to create an immediate atmosphere of being present "right here, right now" to help you rediscover your own humanity and find the new, refreshed beginning of personal happiness and joy.

The Montgomery Model of Heart-to-Heart Resuscitation embraces a personal approach to therapy and counseling. This approach eclipses most conventional therapies in that it focuses on special military needs and dynamics that most civilian clinicians do not encounter in a lifetime. In fact, not many Veteran Affairs doctors, social workers, or nurses specialize in combat veteran psychological trauma. Most have never looked deep into the eyes or heard the cries of the wounded souls. I have been present with them and will tell you it is enough to tear your heart out.

So, how does H2HR work? The journey begins with rigorous peer-based groups that utilize instructional discussions, storytelling, and team-building group activities designed to challenge warriors to overcome their past experiences and move forward into a life of purpose. Heart to heart resuscitation programs allow veterans to appreciate the peace of a secure experience while they focus on their challenges in completing the program.

Two days a week, 90-minute sessions of intensive peer-to-peer group programs serve as the catalyst to help veterans discover the answers to the big questions in life. Challenges related to the struggles of former daily military life, combat deployments. and the symptoms of post-traumatic stress (PTS) surface during an ensuing 18 months of group work. The H2HR program teaches veterans how to identify and fight through challenges that might have been limiting their personal success and family relationships.

The program for men and women is a confidential and open environment that fosters camaraderie and friendship. Utilizing peer relationships, participants find common ground through shared experiences and understanding, allowing a greater potential for growth and recovery. Through developing discipline, team-building skills, courage in embracing a new life, a sense of honor, and love for family, the veterans develop character and learn to live a life of leadership. The H2HR program equips warriors to fight through life's challenges and discover the very purpose for their lives moving forward.

The atmosphere created in and by the group is unique. The H2HR program is safe, confidential, and disarmingly authentic. The group talk is not just presented; it's demonstrated through storytelling. The group opens windows into the participating vets' lives with unbridled honesty, sharing from the heart personal failures as well as new and continuing victories.

Military service breeds a high level of connectedness and community—a brotherhood or sisterhood. Heart to heart resuscitation takes that level of team and pumps it up to new heights. Counselors and participants don't just say, "I've got your six;" they live it. The H2HR program is truly remarkable and must be experienced to fully understand. Group attendance challenges perceptions and changes lives.

## Why is this book needed?

Foundations of trust and a caring attitude are the most fundamental of human needs emotionally crushed vets require and want from their healthcare providers. And is at the very foundation of Heart-to-Heart Resuscitation. A simple, genuine, direct statement, such as "I care you are here today, I care that you get the help you need, or I care about you, buddy," communicated face-to-face or over the phone is a meaningful way to begin an encouraging, caring therapeutic relationship. In my experience, those words are very important and have brought tears to the eyes of many combat-seasoned, the toughest of the tough veterans, who hear them for the first time. The need to reconnect, especially for a combat veteran, is vital for a successful recovery. Warriors in combat have their battle buddies, rifle teams, squads, and rifle team leaders to have their back. When they are discharged, the units usually are broken up, leaving the veteran alone to fight the innermost battles—a daunting task.

The need to feel normal runs deep. "Act normal" is their mantra. Simply processing PTSD combat warriors through the revolving doors as they do cattle in the stockyards heading for slaughter is not the level of mental health care they need or deserve.

My experience over the decades while treating honorable warriors serving in several war zones, suggests that while the war ends our military soldiers and Marines come home facing uncertainty and readjustment to civilian life and family and friends' daily routines once again. The immediate changes can be challenging and stressful.

"Ilona Meagher (2008), editor of the Web site *PTSD Combat*, published the following statistics on Army mental health and suicides in her article "OEF/OIF Veteran Suicide Toll:"

- Nearly 40 percent of Army suicides in 2006 and 2007 were committed by veterans taking psychotropic drugs for depression and PTSD under doctors' orders (CBS News).

- Nearly 60 percent of 948 Army veterans who made suicide attempts in 2006 had been seen by mental health providers before the attempt—36 percent within just 30 days of the event.

- More than 43,000 U.S. troops since 2003 were sent into combat even though they had been listed as medically unfit in the weeks before their scheduled deployment.1

One afternoon, my 2 p.m. appointment, a war hero, told me a story that changed my life forever. We were sitting together in my counseling office. This Marine, a Silver Star recipient, sat up straight as a board on the fully cushioned armchair directly in front of me. Face to face.

"Vic," he said, I have never told what I am going to tell you to anyone, ever. I feel I can trust you buddy. You said you have my six, right?"

"Right," I said emphatically, looking him straight in the eyes.

Tears flowed down his cheeks. I handed him a box of tissues as he sniffled and struggled to talk. "Our rifle team was reinforcing a combat rifle company support base the same day I arrived in Vietnam. Half of us were FNG ( F----G New Guys). The first day we arrived at our base we were under attack by mortar fire, snipers, with VC (Viet Cong) crawling all over the hills like an army of ants. Next thing I knew I was face down in my muddy trench that I earlier had dug with my trenching tool. I was numb. I felt I had an out-of-body life experience. I don't remember much of anything…just explosions and bullets zinging by me, hitting the mud. I was so full of fear and anger I began firing clip after clip. At times, I remember thinking I was flying above the hole, feeling as if my body was floating. What the hell! What was happening? Vic, I never got over that experience. Two of my buddies died that day. I didn't get a scratch, but my emotions are another thing. My heart hurts when I think about the experience and my buddies. I can't get this shit out of my mind. I'm dying here I've got a hole in my heart, Vic."

Dr. Edward Tick (2005), the much-sought-after military psychotherapist and author, would call many veterans in distress as having …"soul wounding and soul loss as authentic conditions." page 16.

I emphatically agree; their souls desperately need revival. The vets need to know they are loved and that someone cares about them. Numerous veterans have psychological issues stemming from lingering childhood and adolescent experiences. Crisis intervention for these veterans is really all about the integration of theology and psychology: spirituality and cognitive behavioral therapy. The process of heart-to-heart resuscitation is active listening, responding with empathy, encouraging, motivating, and mentoring veterans from the heart, not the head. It is all about building trust and genuine care. The buddy system is what kept these warriors alive in the war. So, ideally, the buddy system has a better chance of keeping them alive through their present challenges.

I don't necessarily believe that only service-connected veteran counselors and therapists can do the job, but I do advocate that veterans counseling veterans and clean and sober recovering alcoholics counseling or sponsoring alcoholics will result in more successful outcomes. I do not possess a scientific method or peer-reviewed study to give to your outcome statistics, but I do have over twenty years' experience helping veterans and others find their way.

Please, do not misunderstand me. Much credit for recovery must begiven to dedicated social workers, nurses, therapists, and caregivers within the VA system, but I believe we need to define what it is that warriors need, not what we think is applicable. We must think out of the box when dealing with combat traumatized veterans. I feel the general attitude of heart-to-heart resuscitation is what most wounded souls want and need to hear. Most combat warriors have been emotionally torn, tattered, battered and stressed beyond belief waiting for their vehicles to be hit by roadside blasts or booby traps to explode when kicking in doors of suspected insurgents' hideouts. Many veterans in war zones wear audio headsets in their helmets blasting heavy metal and rap music to motivate them into firefights and seek-and-destroy missions. The high-volume music seems to desensitize the moment.

In general, most vets are tough and well-trained but scared when preparing for combat. It is my belief and experience that wholly effective and genuine substance abuse counselors, nurses, licensed clinical social workers, addiction therapists and treatment team psychologists are born, not made. However, we all can learn from one another's experiences and research. Counselors and therapists choosing to use the H2HR model in the treatment of suicidal veterans must first learn to express genuineness and demonstrate the ability to actively listen, not intellectually pontificate. I believe crisis interventionists and crisis line responders will have the greatest success in veterans' rescues when they own the ability and willingness to feel what the veteran feels and accept every veteran in crisis with unconditional positive regard. By showing acceptance and unconditional positive regard, a counselor provides the best conditions for a client's personal growth.

Psychologist Carl Rogers (1957) introduced the concept of unconditional positive regard[1], defining it as follows:

> "It means caring for the client, but not in a possessive way or in such a way as simply to satisfy the therapist's own needs…. It means caring for the client as a separate person, with permission to have his own feelings, his own experiences."

If the mental health provider or caretaker does not exhibit these beliefs, the veteran's realization for a positive outcome will be minimal, no matter how many reassessment and therapeutic techniques are used. Heart-to-Heart Resuscitation is all about reflective caring. Rogers suggests reflection is the mirroring of emotional communication.

## How can this book be best used?

Throughout this book, I have included examples of action plans and treatment planning. The Montgomery Model of Heart-to-Heart Resuscitation for veteran rescues offers a much more empathetic theory than usually taught in graduate schools. Please, don't misunderstand me. There are many quality and qualified clinicians in the world. However, I have found that combat-hardened veterans come to their clinicians with a special, extreme, highly emotional, and aroused state of mind. Many have been abandoned by the military, their family, and friends, and they are broken-hearted.

---

1. For those who like to follow ideas back to their origins, Rogers (1961), who is widely credited as the innovator of this concept, indicated that the source of his theory came from the work of a graduate student, Stanley Standal, who proposed it in his 1954 dissertation on the same topic.

# CHAPTER 1

# Welcome to Group Room #2
# Where Veterans in Distress Gather

As mentioned in the introduction, Group Room #2 at the clinic where I work the meeting place for veterans looking for help. Joe and his new roommate were among them

When these two first showed up at Group Room #2 for the evening veteran's group, they signed in at the front desk, then found the room, and sat down.

Around 6 p.m., I walked from my office across the hall, entered the group room, and sat down among the dozen vets. No one in the room said much of anything. I, also, sat in silence, briefly looking around and engaging each vet face to face.

Then, I spoke, "Good evening, everyone. I hope you all had a clean and sober week." There were sheepish looks and glares—and a few smiles.

"I would like to introduce the newest member of our group. Please, welcome Joe Ferguson." A few group participants nodded or offered a halfhearted wave. Some just stared at Joe. He stood his ground, giving back "mad dog" stares to those who challenged him with a cold stare.

Joe was streetwise and street-tough. Not much rattled LT Joe Ferguson, especially since he stopped drinking, entered detox, and had been clean for 11 days. He sat steady among the vets in the room, determination on his face.

I continued, "Before Joe shares some of his story with all of you, let's go around the room and introduce yourselves to him. Give your name, why you are here, where and when you served in the military, and what your former specialty or MOS and rank were. Who would like to start?"

I vividly recall looking around the room that day, peering into the faces of many broken, cast-down warriors. The beginning of the long road home had just begun for Joe Ferguson and the 11 others in the room.

"Well, what the hell, Vic. I will start!" Danny popped up, "My name is Danny 81, opiate addict, parolee fresh out of prison for aggravated assault, nearly killed a guy with my knife in a bar fight. Thought I was in the 'Nam'... done 8 years hard time, Sing Sing Prison New York. My parole officer sent me here, saying I need to stop my aggressive behavior and stop using and selling illegal drugs. If I don't come here to get counseling, my PO said, she will violate me and send me back up to the big house... nasty place Sing Sing. They call it a correctional facility. Correctional, my ass! Did you know over 600 people have been executed there, fried until their eyeballs popped out? Some kind of correction, huh?" Danny smirked slightly, paused, and shifted in his chair, his hands gripping the sides of the padded seat. Rigid, with a puzzled and troubled look on his face, he glanced over at me. "What were the other things you wanted me to say counselor?"

"I want you to share with the others in the group what your rank and MOS were and what outfit you served with in combat."

"Oh, yeah, okay." Danny's voice was intense and razor-sharp. "I'm a former 1st Lieutenant US Marine Corps, 0306 MOS, Infantry Weapons Officer, Vietnam Tet Offensive, 1968-69. The VC called us Devil Dogs. It got ugly over there, lots of body bags and ponchos filled with body parts."

As Danny was sharing parts of his story, his face contorted—upper lip snarled and cheeks red. His body stiffened as he revisited battlefield scene flashbacks floating through his mind as he was speaking. He took a breath, then slowly turned his closely trimmed, graying head and bearded face and stared over at Joe. He took a full minute. The silence was penetrating.

I took that opportunity to glance around the circle, observing each face in the room, not saying a thing but watching the eyes and facial expressions and body posture of everyone sitting there that day. The non-verbal communication of the faces and body positions spoke volumes.

Then, staring straight into Joe's eyes from across the room, with a serious expression, Danny broke the silence, "Welcome home, Joe! Oorah!" Joe's upper lip twitched as he just stared back at Danny.

"Thanks for starting us off, Danny. Now, let's continue the introductions counterclockwise around the room." I pointed to Chad Williams, sitting just to the left of Danny Barnes.

I first met Chad Williams just a few days earlier when he told me about his struggles with addiction to pain killers. He was a self-professed "prescription drug junkie and drunk." The 28-year-old Army combat veteran served three tours in Afghanistan, one with Task Force DAGGER in 2001. The vet told me about a flight in a helicopter flying into a mountain landing zone somewhere in Afghanistan, conducted at night in mountains as high as 16,000 feet with clouds, rain, and even sandstorms creating dangerous obstacles. He went on to tell me he was with one of the Special Forces teams that infiltrated into northern Afghanistan. I vividly remember him describing the battlefields: "They moved us over difficult terrain by horse and on foot, infiltrating into the mountains where we first engaged the Taliban on the north side of the pass."

Sergeant Williams had been injured on his last tour in Afghanistan, 2004 when a suicide bomber pulled his truck out onto the road and into the on-coming convoy of Humvees, exploding the first two vehicles. The explosion was so strong Sergeant Williams, riding in the third vehicle, and others received head concussions by the bomb blast impact.

"I was told I was unconscious for almost an hour," he told me. "My medical diagnosis was finally determined to be Moderate Traumatic Brain Injury and Post Traumatic Stress Disorder. I was redeployed stateside and discharged. It was difficult for me to fit in. My family had no idea what I had been through. No one understands unless they were there. I had no visible wounds, but day by day I was dying a slow death inside, invisibly."

Proper treatment and even VA benefits were hard to come by because mild-to-moderate closed-brain injury in the war zone was difficult to identify. Many vets exposed to blasts in Iraq and Afghanistan slipped through the cracks. Debriefing and mental health assessment was limited or non-existent. The processing was slow. Warriors received little or no help when they needed it the most. Combat veterans ended up self-medicating rather than cause a stir at a VA hospital in trying to be seen for an injury few clinicians understood. Chad shared he continued to experience confusion, migraines and headaches, trouble sleeping, some nightmares, and disturbing dreams reliving the traumatic bombing and other fire-fight experiences in country. Dismembered bodies, blood, and guts peppered his memories.

He also expressed that. along with feelings of hopelessness and helplessness, he experienced anxiety and depression, including some thoughts of ending his life. Chad told me he had a plan to kill himself on several occasions.

"Vic, no one ever asked me about suicidal thoughts or attempts, and no military doctor ever referred me to a treatment center for drug abuse. In fact, they asked very little about my drinking habits."

I clearly remember Chad saying to me, "The doctors in the war zone would only write scripts for Benzodiazepines and antidepressants to treat me—no therapy or counseling to help my mind. The drugging all started in the war, in the Army."

It has been my years of experience and accretion of knowledge while learning ever more about Traumatic Brain Injury that most combat warriors exposed to these types of blast wave explosions will fully recover within a few weeks. On the other hand, a lesser percentage will never recover and will continue to experience debilitating symptoms, leaving them unable to fully interact with their families, friends or hold a job.

Such was the case with Chad Williams. He self-medicated, drinking alcoholically and using other drugs, including opioids (Oxycodone). Most of the time he would find non-VA doctors to offer him nerve pills and sedative prescriptions. When he could not get a prescription refill from a doctor, he would buy pills on the street illegally or offshore.

It is well known by most substance abuse processionals that prolonged use of Benzos is not recommended and can result in physical and mental dependency as well as severe withdrawal symptoms. Chad had found that out the hard way. He was unable to cope any longer. He claimed he had hit his proverbial bottom. The self-medication did not work for him anymore. So, here he was in group room #2.

"I'm Chad Williams trying to get off the booze and pain killers and other prescription drugs ever since combat in Afghanistan 2001. I served in Army Special Forces, Sergeant, three tours. We got our ass kicked by a suicide bomber, who blew up our convoy. I have a concussion head injury; my best buddy lost his legs. It was nasty! Now, my older brother, my best friend, checked me into the clinic a few days ago, said I need help and can't hang around his house anymore until I get treatment and stop drinking. He said I have changed and am scaring his wife and the kids. I don't think he even knows I am popping pills, too."

Chad choked up, then cleared his throat. His head bobbed and weaved, looking around the room, trying to solicit some understanding. "I can't even hold a stinking job. I'm too unreliable, they say. It's over for me," His voice elevated, "Shit, I don't know why I'm even here. I 'm a dead man walking!" With that, Chad leaped up out of his chair, heading for the door. "F--k me…it's over, man!"

I stood up immediately, side stepping to block his way out of the room, but did not put my hands on him, trying to show a team spirit of support. Just then, another warrior from the group jumped up and stepped in next to Chad— Jimmy Maxwell, U.S. Army Airborne. Jimmy reached out and laid his hand on Chad's right shoulder while he uttered under his breath, "Hey, buddy, I've got your back. We are all in this together. Oorah!"

What Jimmy Maxwell did that evening was a huge first step in building support and cohesiveness within the veteran group. In battle, the buddy system is everything. It is a matter of life and death on many fronts. The buddy system is encouraged in the Army and Marines during basic training and continues into battle. The advantages have been found to increase morale, decrease stress, encourage, motivate, and developed confidence. The buddy system is an integral part and necessity to increasing the odds of staying alive and improving safety for one another while in a firefight.

And so, it is also in group counseling. Recovery from chemical dependency addiction is also a life and death battle. Support, motivation, and encouragement are key elements in helping each other break through the overwhelming barriers that confront every alcoholic and addict. Make no mistake, the out-of-control consumption of alcohol and other types of drugs is 100% lethal. The unsuspecting user is guaranteed a death sentence—by suicide, accidental overdose, physical or mental collapse or death caused by violence. Guaranteed!

Chad took a moment, looking at Jimmy and then at me. The angry soldier went back to his padded chair and sat down. He instantly looked down at his feet, leaning slightly forward, elbows on his knees, fists clinched. The room was filled with a strained stillness.

Once again, I glanced around the room, taking in the pain, puzzled faces of the vets who knew it would soon be their turn to talk. I looked in the direction of both female veterans, one just to the left of Chad: Alice Anderson, heroin addict, Reserve Army Nurse, Afghanistan, 3D Medical Command, Operation Enduring Freedom 2002.

Normally, in the veteran groups I have facilitated in the last decade, there has always been a low percentage of women enrolled. Sometimes, veteran women do not attend at all. I can find this is in government and independent reports indicating that of the 220,00 or so women in the military, only a few serve in direct combat missions. Most of the military women are reported to serve in support roles: communications, healthcare, logistics officers, and so on—albeit the numbers assigned to combat are increasing every year. So, when there are women in the groups, I stand by for fireworks.]

"You're up, Alice," I announced. "Welcome to group." I looked around the circle, and everyone was staring at one of only two females in the room. *This must be intimidating and uncomfortable,* I remember thinking.

Alice's shiny, dyed-black hair was pulled tight into a ponytail with a thick, red ribbon. Her piercing, dark-green eyes were hard to resist. This 33-year-old military nurse veteran appeared ready to take on all comers. Her aging, high-cheek-boned face maintained the beauty of a Native American heritage. Her full lips were lined with a deep-red lipstick, matching the ribbon in her hair. She wore tight, faded, blue-jean overalls with a flowered, long sleeve shirt and collar revealing a busty cleavage.

As Alice prepared to talk, she sat straight up in her chair without a moment of hesitation. Her aging, veined hands were folded on her lap. Alice had turned into one tough customer, learning to live in the world of wounded and dismembered soldiers and heroin addicts.

In a throaty voice, Alice Anderson began talking. She first looked hard into the gawking faces of the guys in the room. "Don't, for a minute, you assholes, think you are going to get close to this…yeah…I know, some of you will want to touch this booty or be my big brother and all that shit. Don't even think about it."

The straight-faced nurse turned her head to look at me. "My name is Alice Anderson, heroin addict, seven days clean. I enlisted in the Army Reserve in 2000, fresh out of community college. I went into nursing and ended up as a Reserve Army Nurse. I was sent over to the war, Operation Enduring Freedom. We nurses were called "desert medics." among other things. I was assigned to a surgical team as a practical nurse. Our field medical unit moved quickly into battles like Operation Anaconda—lots of blood and guts."

Chad Williams spoke up loudly, "Shit, lady, I was there in 2001 and 2, Special Forces. Hell, I know the blood and guts. I lost a buddy in that Op. You might have worked on him… f--k… ain't that a bitch?"

He just starred at her with ice-cold eyes. Then, he looked over at me and then down at the floor, shaking his head. Alice said nothing more.

"Thanks for sharing, Alice… and Chad, we can revisit what you just shared at another time. Are you okay with that, buddy?"

Chad didn't look up. Alice was fidgeting with her hair and leaning back in her chair, her head tilted back against the wall. She looked up at the ceiling and closed her eyes, lips tightly pressed together. Tears filled the corners of her eye sockets. I moved on.

Sitting just to the left of Alice was Corporal Jared Murdock. "Your turn Mr. Murdock."

Jared was a big farm boy—looked like he could carry 2-, 3-string hay bales on his shoulders at the same time. I always expected to see him come into the clinic with a piece of straw hanging out of the corner of his mouth. He seemed like a gentle giant when I first met him in the clinic waiting room. When I shook his hand, it was like putting on a glove. My hand disappeared.

I recall when Jared first walked into our clinic a couple of years after he was honorably discharged from the Marine Corps. He indicated he had served two consecutive 13-month tours with the 1st Marine Division, 1st Battalion, and 5th Marines-Operation Iraqi Freedom. His job: warrior. His mission: scouting the dangerous roads for insurgents and killing them.

I clearly remember him sharing this information with me, in detail, during our private counseling sessions and group encounters. He had been prescribed antidepressants by the Navy doctors while in the war zone because he was unable to sleep, suffering from unrelenting battle fatigue, anxiety, and depression. He had told me that many of the men in his rifle squad had to be medicated to continue their assault missions. There were no replacement rifle teams coming. He shared that there were times when their search-and-destroy rifle team didn't sleep for several consecutive days while in persistent pursuit of an elusive enemy. Jared told me he was 'hooked' on antidepressants, needing them to function every day in Iraq and to cope with the anxiety and stress of combat. He felt depressed most of the time toward the end of his tour. I recall him saying, "I felt hopeless. I saw no relief in sight."

Jared was referred to me by a local community hospital mental health clinician who knew I was the outpatient clinic's addiction specialist primarily counseling combat veterans in the area. The referral report passed on to me indicated Jared was found by friends sitting in the dark of another friend's apartment, rambling to himself, acting bewildered and disoriented, and experiencing the sensation of insects crawling under his skin.

At the time Jared first came to see me, and after lab drug screening and assessments, he self-disclosed his uncontrollable use of methamphetamines. Apparently, as the story was told, when the Marine sergeant discharged stateside some buddies getting out with him, they introduced him to snorting meth for a more immediate relief from the gloominess and depression he was experiencing. He was buying the stimulant illegally on the streets in the cities and towns around his farming community.

Methamphetamine abusers can display several psychotic features, including paranoia, visual and auditory hallucinations, and delusions. Chronic methamphetamine abuse significantly changes how the brain functions. Noninvasive human brain imaging studies have shown alterations in the activity of the dopamine system that are associated with reduced motor skills and impaired verbal learning. Recent studies in chronic methamphetamine abusers have also revealed severe structural and functional changes in areas of the brain associated with emotion and memory, which may account for many of the emotional and cognitive problems I observed while evaluating Jared.

I recall vividly a "rush" Jared reported, describing his feelings when first using meth as an intense euphoria. Those feelings, he explained, relieved him from the thoughts of the culture shock he experienced when first posted to Iraq and the blood and guts of his war experiences.

He could not forget the order his fire team got to move back out and collect the mutilated enemy dead after a nighttime firefight and discovering that some of the blooded bodies were still alive. "It was ugly," I remember him saying. "And you don't always know who the bad guys are. Which one is going to cut my throat when my back is turned, dragging the bodies away?"

Another discussion stands out for me as well. Jared described the first time he kicked in a door of a small house in Baghdad, searching for terrorists. As he entered the house in a crouched and ready-to-kill position, the first thing he saw lying right in front of him on the dirt floor was a baby doll, toys, kid's shoes, and clothing spread around. The culture shock was unbearable for this farm boy. His first thought was, "What happened to these innocent children?" Jared later told me things like that started affecting him a lot more than he thought they would.

He spoke up, "I don't have much to say. My name is Jared Murdock I served two tours with the 1st Marine Division, 1st Battalion, and 5th Marines in Operation Iraqi Freedom as an 0311 Corporal E-4 rifle team leader." He paused, looking at me for help. I said nothing, acknowledging him only with the nod of my head.

He continued, "We would patrol the booby-trapped, sniper-infested roads and back streets of Iraq searching for insurgents."

He suddenly stopped talking and looked up at the ceiling, rubbing his head with both hands, his palms massaging his eyes. Then, he looked back at me, his voice more controlled, and went on, "Our mission was to search and destroy the enemy: and we did just that. Things got messy. I kicked in hundreds of doors and windows, shit like that. Some of you know what I'm talking about. I saw a lot of shit I can't forget. I think I 'm losing my f--king mind. I'm done. That's it, Vic." Jared immediately leaned back, tilting his chair against the wall and closing his eyes.

I took the lead. "Thanks for sharing, Jared. We can revisit some of those issues at another time, okay?" Jared did not open his eyes. He just raised his left hand limply, raising his thumb, acknowledging his answer.

Slumped down in his chair just to the left of Jared sat Jimmy Maxwell, a rugged, muscular fellow, wearing a faded, sandy brown colored Army Airborne tee shirt with a pattern of sweat stains around the sagging collar and under his armpits. Other vets' similar posture told me a break was needed.

"Good work, everyone. Let's take a 15-minute break. Bathrooms are around the corner to the right. Bottled water, fresh fruit, and cookies are in the kitchen to the left. Come back to the seats you are in now. We will begin with Jimmy Maxwell when we get back."

As I spoke, Jimmy was smiling at me. He had a wide grin and mouth full of chewing tobacco-stained teeth. In fact, the stains from years of chewing chew spilled out of the corners of his mouth.

At the break, I walked straight to my office down the hallway and closed the door. My office was comfortable and welcoming—and safe. My oak desk and credenza were set back against the wall, allowing room for a conversation space with a small couch and two stuffed cushion chairs. Along the wall behind the couch, a long, narrow table supported a decorated stone-and-pebble waterfall lamp, which gave off a soft light and soothing sound of rippling water.

I paused for a moment in that space. I sat down on one of the cushioned chairs and began reflecting about the hundreds of hours I had spent within these walls, helping, encouraging, and motivating so many clients over the years with the desire to always counsel from my heart.

Break was over. We all gathered back in Group Room 2 and sat down.

"Jimmy, it's your turn," I said, looking at him directly.

Jimmy wasn't smiling now. He began looking around the room, speaking in a low tone. "My name is Jimmy Maxwell. Corporal. Served in the Army's 1st Battalion of the 325th Airborne Infantry Regiment in Al-Fallujah, Iraq in 2003, an absolute hellhole. I'm a 34-year-old former paratrooper. Did my share of killing and blowing things up in the sandbox. This isn't my first rodeo. I can't seem to be able to keep the plug in the jug." Jimmy took a breath, wiping his mouth with the back of his hand and bending down and adjusting the laces of his old, desert tan military boots.

This was his first time at our clinic. He had failed to complete four other alcohol and drug treatment programs over the last six years, but he kept coming back for help. Alcohol addiction challenged him. Many alcoholics find themselves relapsing, time after time, before the light switch finally goes on. For some, it never does.

Still bent over his Army boots, Jimmy looked up toward me. "Vic, got to do it this time, counselor, don't think I have another run in me," He looked back down at the floor and continued, "These boots have seen lots of stuff I've held on to for years since I was in country…shared with nobody…told nobody. Got to get it out of my mind, Vic. Nightmares in technicolor, shit like that. That's all I got for now. Next up."

"Good work, Jimmy, and yes, we will work on all that shit," I said in an affirmative, endorsing way. "Right, group?" Several in the group showed support by nodding their heads, and a couple acknowledged in the military fashion, "oorah" or "ooah," depending upon in which branch of the service they had served.

Jimmy sat back in his chair and continued to look in my direction. I looked to his left, where Marine Corporal Garcia sat clenching his teeth and wringing his hands while "mad dogging" the other veterans in group room 2. It was his turn to speak.

Fresh out of detox, the former Marine was still suffering from the withdrawal effects of methamphetamine dependence. He looked abnormally thin—sunken cheeks shiny with sweat. The 34-year-old Ruben smiled nervously, evincing some strain, as he introduced himself.

"I'm a former Marine 0311 'grunt.' Fought over in Iraq, Gulf War, 2003. We kicked the Republican Guard's ass. I was on the front lines with the 1st Marine Division when shit hit the fan. Now, sometimes I can't go anywhere without feeling like those m-f-ers are chasing me. I use whatever drugs I can get my hands on to survive the flashbacks, mostly crystal meth, been living on the streets of East Los Angeles. I'm on parole. My PO told me I must come here or go to prison. That's it."

Ruben remained stiff in his seat, positioned to take on all comers—genuine machismo. Surviving the Iraq War, the invasion of Baghdad, as a Marine rifleman and now living on the mean streets of East LA tells most of his story.

"Okay, Ruben, We will help you get through this tough time in your life. Just let me know what you need for your PO to keep you compliant, and I will make every effort to make sure it gets done—with your help." I looked squarely into Corporal Garcia's eyes and said gruffly, "Oorah!" Ruben starred right back at me as intensely and responded, "Oorah!_--and managed a smile.

Continuing around the room counterclockwise, to the left of Ruben, a female fighter pilot, Lieutenant Bonnar—Hanna—sat straight in her chair, back firmly planted against the chair padding almost as if in the cockpit of one of her fighter jets. Her brunette hair hung short, dangling straight down and tucked over her ears. She wore an interesting lipstick color, light grayish purple, with matching, dangling earrings. Clad in a tan, baggy jumpsuit and soft leather, shiny, ankle-high boots, she appeared fragile and nervous.

I greeted her, "Welcome, Hanna, nice seeing you tonight. If you will, please share a bit of who you are, what units you served in, where your combat took place, and why you are here tonight."

"Sure thing, Vic, I am a veteran, an Air Force combat pilot. My name is Hanna Bonnar," she began in an unsteady voice, and then went on to share she was a combat bomber pilot at the beginning of Operation Desert Storm, an offensive campaign that was originally designed to enforce the United Nation's resolutions that Iraq must cease its rape and pillage of its weaker neighbor Kuwait and withdraw its forces from the small country. She further shared, "Now, at my house, the last couple of years, fireworks have been too much for me".

Though Hanna took prescribed medication from the VA daily, storms, sonic booms from the F-14 jets at the nearby Air Force Base, and almost anything noisy or sudden startled her. The Independence Day fireworks' loud bangs and whistles over and near her house triggered her past experiences as a bomber pilot.

"Too many memories and flashbacks," she said and began to weep. There was a pause of silence as she wiped her eyes. "Sorry," she apologized, quietly looking over my way. Then, clearing her throat, she continued in a whisper, "H-hour, when the air campaign began and until the end of offensive combat operations 43 days later, I helped obliterate key targets, ensuring the United States military and its coalition partners owned the skies over Iraq and Kuwait." She looked around the room, wiping her forehead with the palms of her hands and then wiping them on the top of her pant legs, and then glared at me. For the first time, I noticed her piercing hazel eyes.

She said, "Vic, I have had to learn to live with this painful memory and the thought I could be responsible for the deaths of innocent people, women, and children. My thoughts are intense at times. I feel irritable, and I can't concentrate. I experience life-like daydreams of certain scary experiences that return repeatedly and haunt me; and oh my…the nightmares. I can't take this anymore.," she said with a keen sense of sadness.

"All right. Thank you for sharing, Hanna…some tough stuff." The rest of the group signaled support for her.

"How are you feeling right now, Hanna? Are you okay? Do you need to talk with me after group and process some of the reactions?"

"No, Vic. I will be all right. Thinking of those experiences as I was talking just triggered me. Thank you all for listening. This is why I am her—to work through all of this and learn how to deal with it."

Suddenly, Alice jumped up and crossed the room toward Hanna, Reaching out, she put an arm around Hanna's shoulder, patting her on the back in a reassuring gesture. Then, she returned to her chair. Hanna thanked her.

Sitting to the left of Hanna was Joe Mendez, one of the more seasoned warriors in the room. He fought in the Vietnam War: bloody boots and body bags! His chair was tilted back against the wooden chair rail, his legs crossed with arms folded tightly under his chest. Just by observing Joe's mannerisms and physical appearance, you knew he was a badass, even at his age. Faded ink on his forearm was his calling card: 3rd Marine Sniper Platoon with crosshairs and a skull.

"Joe, your turn, buddy."

Now, Joe's elbows were in the air, hands rubbing his balding head of short gray hair, face distorted as if forcing a thought from deep within his inner sanctum. "My name is Joe Mendez; age 59 years old. Got out of the Corps as a Sergeant E-5, scout sniper, 3rd Marines. Vietnam 1970."

As he finished introducing himself, Joe tilted his chair forward, slowly planting his feet on the floor, and scowled boldly at me from across the room. "Speed balling is the curse God put on my life Vic," he barked out.

Joe was so filled with pent-up emotions that he literally spit with rage when he spoke. He clarified in plain words his use of the lethal mixture called a speedball, the full effects of mixing heroin and cocaine. Then, he continued, "You know, back in Vietnam we all thought we were supermen, indestructible, especially as snipers. And we were young, in our 20s. No fear. So, when I got my first confirmed kill, it was a VC riding a bicycle on the Ho Chi Minh Trail.

I remember like it was yesterday, looking through my scope on my Winchester 70 and squeezing the trigger. I saw his head explode and vaporize like a crushed watermelon. *Now I was officially in the hunt,* I thought. So, why am I here today? It's a long story—a lot of haunting memories—some not so good."

Joe began looking down at his arm ink, pushing at it with his index finger. He paused, looking around the room, then continued, "My wife told me I needed to get help for my nightmares and anger outbursts. If I did not check myself into a clinic to get counseling help, I needed to move out of the house. So, here I am. That's it."

I was watching Joe carefully. I waited to make sure he was alright, then moved on.

All the years I have spent personally mentoring and counseling combat veterans I have known that it's a well kept secret that a significant percentage of combat troops in the war zones are medicated with psychiatric drugs to continue their stressful, deadly missions. In fact, psychiatric drugs are being prescribed, consumed, shared, and traded in combat zones, and many warriors then return stateside chemically dependent on those antipsychotic, anti-anxiety drugs and sleeping pills.[2]

Sergeant Russ Mason was no exception. He, too, had trouble getting to sleep and calming his post-traumatic stress and was prescribed psychiatric drugs. Russ came into the clinic and needed help learning to relax enough to be able to readjust to civilian life back home–without drugs.

"Yeah ... my name is Russ Mason, 42 years old, Sergeant... Marine Sergeant, 1st Armored Division, Machine Gunner, Desert Storm, Gulf War."

Russ slowly looked around the room, then at me, and added, "Returning home and readjusting, looking for a job, and everyday family routines suck! And on top of all that shit, the docs tell me I am addicted to the same type of drugs they gave me in the Corps—the same shit they gave me for years. Ain't that a bitch!"

---

2. As early as 2009, NBC reported, "According to data from a U. S. Army mental-health survey released last year, about 12 percent of soldiers in Iraq and 15 percent of those in Afghanistan reported taking antidepressants, anti-anxiety medications, or sleeping pills. Prescriptions for painkillers have also skyrocketed. Data from the Department of Defense last fall showed that as of September 2007, prescriptions for narcotics for active-duty troops had risen to almost 50,000 a month, compared with about 33,000 a month in October 2003, not long after the Iraq war began."

Russ looked snappishly over toward Alice and said awkwardly, "Excuse my French, Alice." Alice nodded her head slightly, expressing forgiveness—with a sheepish smile.

Sergeant Mason continued looking at me directly while sharing his introduction, "Been in the Corps eight plus years, Vic, and just transferred from the VA last month." The Sergeant restlessly readjusted his position on his padded stacking chair every couple of minutes, remaining visibly engaged with another vet in the room, starring at him with a laser-sharp glare until the other warrior lost the contest and looked away.

In country, Russ Mason had been a machine gunner in a Marine Armored Division in Iraq with direct orders to search and destroy the enemy, the insurgents, and the Republican Guard tank divisions. The challenge every day for Russ was figuring out what the enemy looked like and to differentiate between the good guys and the bad guys. They all looked like bad guys. So, every day in the war zones, in the sandboxes, contained a new set of stressors for the gunner: to fight, engage, or observe? For months at a time, Russ faced many hidden obstacles every day, which resulted in a constant state of hyper vigilance and anxiety. He would contemplate: What's it going to be today? Improvised Explosive Devises (IED) or incoming from enemy tanks and military vehicles and armor piercing shells? Or would he and his team be exposed to snipers dug in on the rooftops or rocket propelled grenades whistling overhead? In Russ's mind, day in and day out, were thoughts of how to keep his tank safe from enemy fire. The pressure for a gunner was always on.

Since getting out, Russ had been suffering from hyper vigilance symptoms and had become preoccupied with constantly scanning his environment around him for possible threats, causing him to lose connections with his family and friends. Just walking down the street in his neighborhood, Russ might overreact to loud and unexpected noises or become agitated in highly crowded or noisy settings. He would often have a difficult time getting to sleep or staying asleep. Sustained states of hyper vigilance, lasting for a decade or more, led to higher sensitivity to disturbances and an inability to tolerate very small or large groups. In such cases, people become exhausted after constantly having to resolve these issues and are often unable to function in normal society.

"It's not easy," Russ continued. "I have been having a hard time getting close to my wife and others in the family...my kids. So many years of being a warrior has taken something from me. I look at things differently. I'm just tryin' to get some of my old self back. I'm hoping some of you can understand the shit I'm goin' through." Russ stopped talking abruptly and looked at me as if asking for help. A few others in the group acknowledged his plight with expressive up-and-down head bobs and a couple "Oorahs!"

Suddenly, Jimmy Maxwell jumped up out of his seat and quickly shuffled across the floor, left arm extended toward Russ, fist clinched, soliciting a fist bump. Russ immediately without hesitation raised his right arm with clenched fist and drilled a reciprocal bump, saying, "Thanks, man." Jimmy, all smiles, then spun around and returned to his chair.

I immediately responded, "Russ, welcome home, Sergeant. You are in the right place. We as a group will be here for you. Thank you for sharing."

Sitting just to the left of Sergeant Mason was Army Corporal Tony Cellino. Tony was a tall, wiry character, looking a bit awkward at times but with a warm inviting smile. "Tony, your turn buddy."

Tony slid forward in his chair, both hands holding the chrome sides of the seat frame as if keeping his balance. At first, he stared at his feet, just nodding his head. Slowly, he looked up at me, tears rolling down his high, chiseled cheekbones. His eyelids drooped like a sad puppy. The pain and anguish he was feeling inside was written on his face.

"I can't right now," Tony sobbed lowly while looking back down at the floor.

I immediately jumped in. reaching over and picking up a box of tissues from the side table and handing them to him. "Okay, Tony, we are here for you buddy. We have your back. Take your time. We can come back to you at another time."

I saw at this moment it was important for me to help Tony reduce his stress and anxiety. So, I decided to have him do a relaxation breathing exercise. I pulled my chair over in front of this wounded warrior and said in a low and measured tone, "Tony, take a moment and take a deep breath to help you relax ...ready..." Tony was looking directly into my eyes. "Now, sit back, feet flat on the floor. Breathe in through your nose. Hold it for a moment. Then, exhale through your mouth. Okay, good. Again, slowly, in through the nose. Hold it a couple of seconds. Good. Then, out through the mouth."

Success! Corporal Cellino was beginning to relax, showing signs of steady breathing, and wiping his nose and eyes with the tissues. I moved my chair back against the wall and sat down.

Tony is a 27-year-old, US. Army Corporal, 10th Mountain Division, 3rd Brigade Combat Team and was on a mission when he sustained injuries in a roadside bombing. He was rapidly deployed stateside to undergo surgery. Tony understood first-hand what addiction to narcotic pain killer medicine was all about.

As I settled back into my chair in Group Room 2, I checked in with everyone in the group to see how they felt about what just had happened with Tony. "How is everyone? Some tough stuff, right? We all must deal with suppressed emotions. So, the lesson learned today is how to relax when we become overwhelmed. Just like Tony did with his breathing. It helped settle him down. Right, Tony?"

Tony gave me a thumbs-up, and I continued, "We will come back to you, Tony, as soon as you feel up to sharing a little bit about yourself. Okay, buddy?" Tony nodded.

"Well, let's continue around the room. Sergeant Smith, you are next."

There were no smiles on this rugged Top Sergeant's clean-shaven face today. Top's body was thick, head to toe. He wore a starched, light-green, long-sleeved shirt, faded jeans, and a "spit-shined" pair of boots. In fact, he looked like he could be ready for a "junk-on-the-bunk" Marine Corps barracks inspection at any time.

Marine Gunnery Sergeant James "Smitty" Smith has been a part of the 3/3 since 1983 when the 3rd Battalion, 3rd Marines deployed off the coast of Lebanon for several weeks during a particularly tense period in the civil war. He deployed again in 1990 as part of Operation Desert Shield and saw action at the Battle of Khafji—and again during the liberation of Kuwait. In 2004, he once again deployed overseas in support of Operation Enduring Freedom in Afghanistan and in 2006 and 2007 to Iraq.

Smitty is a distinguished Marine platoon leader. His fighting units have been awarded Presidential Unit Citations for gallantry. The quintessence of Esprit de Corps, the 59-year-old, retired veteran is addicted to uppers and downers. Uppers give you extra energy, primarily by robbing your reserves. They keep you awake when your body really would rather be sleeping. Downers send you to sleep and tend to numb your feelings and lower your sensitivity. They are therefore used to escape from the pains and problems of life.

"My name is Jim Smith. You can all call me Smitty. My life sucks. I have no purpose, no reason for living. What the hell, I get up in the morning and go to bed at night. Retirement sucks. What the hell is that! They put you out to pasture to die. I guess you can call me a war hero with the 3/3, but what do you do with that at the end of the day? I guess my problem, and why I am here, as I see it is I am a warrior of many battles, but now the battles have come home to roost. I am fighting for my life, and I can't find my way. In the Corps, at least my buddies had my back. Now, I must go it alone."

Just then, a slow roll of muffled "oorahs" and "ooahs" filled the room. I looked at Smitty for a moment, then around the room, and smiled and said, "Hey, Top, it appears to me you've got your team back." Gunnery Sergeant Smith looked down at the floor, shaking his head up and down, obviously moved by the moment, and reciprocated to the group with a guttural, "Oorah!"

"Well, Bill, it is your turn before we hear from our newest member, Joe. You're up!"

"Yeah, my name is Bill Foreman Army medic, age 66. Served with the 54th Medical Detachment, 'Dust Off Missions' in 1965, Chu Lai, Vietnam."

Bill's gray-bearded face was contorted, a vein in the side of his neck bulging as he began searching for words to share with the group. Both of his lanky arms, covered with colorful tattoo ink, settled in on his lap as he began to speak.

"They gave me an M14 rifle and .45 pistol, but hell under fire, trying to stop the bleeding of a wounded soldier, how the hell could I defend myself? I needed both hands in the wound. Shit! Bullets were whistling by my head and mortars exploding all around. It was ugly, man. I can't get it out of my head. After all this time, I still feel the fear. Our helicopter was bullet-riddled, and the bay was soaked with blood. One big nightmare, man. Guys were dying in my arms as body parts were missing. Who wouldn't need drugs to get through that? I had an unlimited supply of morphine. So, here am I." Doc stopped talking and studied the faces in the room staring at him. Many looked away or down at the floor in silence. You could hear a pin drop.

Army medic, Doc Foreman had found a haven. Morphine is a narcotic pain reliever prescribed to treat moderate to severe pain, but it also gives an abuser a false sense of well-being. When morphine is abused, an addiction can form very rapidly.

After a moment, I looked at Joe Ferguson. He was sitting straight up in his chair, rubbing his upper thighs with his hands. "Okay, Joe, you have met the group and got a little information about each one of them. Now, it is your turn. Please, introduce yourself."

Joe was sitting next to me dressed in casual clothing and a worn-leather flight jacket. He looked comfortable and unassuming while he began to speak. "I'm a former Navy pilot. My name is Joe Ferguson. I am 48 years old. Served in the Persian Gulf War. Back in the day I trained in the United States Navy Fighter Weapons School at Naval Air Station Miramar in California, known as TOPGUN."

Lieutenant Ferguson is a decorated navy pilot and combat veteran. In combat he was skilled, confident, and powerful. Today, he felt dead inside. He knew he must be in hell. Joe's gut-wrenching account epitomizes the horrific struggles combat warriors face returning home from war zones, addicted to alcohol and other drugs. Joe used alcohol to numb the graphic nightmares and flashbacks he suffered, reliving his bombing sorties on the "Highway of Death" in the Persian Gulf.

Joe continued as he looked around the room, "Alcohol is kicking my ass, That's why I am here. You would think a navy pilot 'Top gun' officer would be able to handle his booze and processing the war zone carnage. After all, that is what I signed up to do as a fighter pilot, right? Hell, no! Not even close! We were blowing up civilian vehicles along with the bad guys. How do you sleep at night with those images flying around in your head night after night?"

Joe stopped talking and looked at me. "Vic, I'm bushed for today. Will share more at another time. Okay?"

I acknowledged Joe, "Thank you for sharing, Joe," then looked into the faces of the other vets in the room and said "And all of you, great work! That will be it for tonight. Good work everyone. Just a reminder … I have individual counseling appointments with each one of you the rest of this week. See me before you leave if there are any questions."

I stood up, made my way to the door, and opened it. I greeted all the vets in the room as they filed out. No one said a word. Then, after the last one exited, I left the room and slowly walked to my office and closed the door.

The next week and second evening in group room # 2, I stood in front of my chair next to Lieutenant Joe Ferguson and began looking around the room, engaging each vet face to face, Then, I began to speak,

"Welcome back. I am hoping you have come to our veteran's group meeting tonight with a purpose in mind. I ask you, what are you looking to accomplish, what is your goal? Well, my desire is that you are looking for *hope* and a healed and renewed future. Please, be aware you are not alone in this battle to understand the meaning of your life and purpose. Today, your mind and heart may feel overwhelmed, especially after combat war trauma experiences that are too difficult to talk about. I congratulate you on your courage to want to change."

Silent desperation stared back at me. I sat down and continued.

"Let us examine for a moment the action plan I am proposing for each one of you as it pertains to your *mind, heart,* and *soul.* Let me explain. The action of the *mind* creates a linking of logic and ration because languages use words to compute or understand, develop intelligence, and talk. Generally, the mind is referred to as a processor of information. Wouldn't you all agree?" I took a minute to let the group reflect. No one spoke.

I continued, "Now, the idea of examining your *heart* is a concept that links together many other concepts such as emotions, feelings, or impulses. Generally, this is understood to be a connection, originating in the 'heart' and being symbolic of life, living, and vitality, right? Most important, your heart serves as your energy source, Does that make sense to you?"

Several in the group were nodding their heads up and down in agreement. Others looked on with puzzled, inquiring faces.

I smiled and continued, "and finally, think about this as your action relates to your *soul,* it involves the mental capabilities of you as a living human being, used for reason, character, feeling, and consciousness. The soul is our intellectual power. Soul is generally defined as the essence of that person. An example of your soul is the part of you that makes you who you are, your real self, your character, and your feelings."

"Does any of this make sense to you?" I paused, looking into the face of each vet.

I felt so much emotion in the air. It was hard to explain. It was tense. No words were spoken. The expression on the faces of the veterans told their stories.

I leaned forward and continued, "I am hoping each one of you will be able to understand more about how this will apply to your lives as time goes on and the more group discussions you attend and writing you get done in your journals."

Changing focus a bit, I continued, "Now, I would like to talk to you for a moment about how you process pain and trauma. This should be helpful to you as you navigate through your healing process. Pain is a great teacher. Yet, the greatest teacher imparts little wisdom if we have not eyes to see and the ears to hear. A helpful way to address this concern is to consider the following spiritual assumptions about trauma and pain:"

"I would like to quote a distinguished therapist and author who once wrote:

> I write this so that we may benefit from our suffering and triumph over our pain… and in the process become better, stronger, warmer, more compassionate, deeper, happier human beings—realizing that the ultimate value of pain reduction is not comfort, but growth. (Glenn R. Schiraldi, PhD (2000)"

I paused, looked around the room, and then continued speaking, "So, if we don't work through the emotions around trauma and stress, they will gradually 'eat us up' to the point where many aspects of our lives will be negatively impacted forever. The moment to change is now. not tomorrow. Tomorrow never gets here. Learning to live in the present is an all-important goal toward living a more peaceful life. We are all unavoidably victims of time to some degree because a rapid rate of living has become the norm in our fast-paced, highly motivated, and highly-strung society. For this reason, it is important that we understand that to not be present is to be torn between two worlds, the past and the future, neither of which exist. To constantly reside in this state prevents us from enjoying life and finding happiness. If you allow yourself to be a victim of time—a victim of the past war experiences and a slave to a future that is yet to unravel—you will carry with you a sense of anxiety. You will be susceptible to stress, agitation and a general discomfort with life. There is no redemption to be found in past or future time. So, surrender to what is right now. Wherever you are, commit to being there, completely. Life will take care of the rest. Hold on for the ride! We will be discussing more about learning how to live 'in the present' in the weeks to come."

I paused, looking at each vet, then continued, "The only requirement to attend this veterans' group is the desire and willingness to change your negative thinking and self-destructive behavior. If you are open and willing to listen to me and the other veterans in this room and follow the stages of recovery I am suggesting—helping heal your mind, heart and soul—you are off to a great start."

No one said a word. Most just stared at me in silence.

"Let's begin tonight talking about first things first: making the commitment, finding a purpose, and applying a plan of action. How does that sound to you?"

I looked around the room. There were muffled grunts and half-hearted mumbling in the circle, but no one spoke a word. Many just looked at their feet, and some had the thousand-mile stare; but no opposition—that night.

I began explaining, "We must first admit that our war zone experiences are troubling and unmanageable to us. The combat is over, yet we continue to struggle mentally, emotionally, and spiritually. Right? In fact, most of us share a common thread of experiences, having the same bad memories over and over, not wanting to get close to anyone, numbing out, wanting to be alone, becoming angry and full of rage at the drop of a hat, and having trouble sleeping. At times, many of us experience muscles becoming tight and tense and having a sense of panic shoot through our very being. Sound familiar? We have difficulty concentrating and often feel confused, sad, frightened, limp, and depressed. Most of the time, as veteran warriors, we mistrust others and frequently look over our shoulders—nobody there to have our back. We feel alone now. Finally, we hold on to massive feelings of guilt about surviving the war when so many of our buddies were lost. Let's take a closer look.

I will be going over the first question for you to think about tonight, and your answers will be part of the beginning of developing your treatment plan. We will be going over your personal plan in our one-on one individual counseling sessions and discussing what you are willing to share here in group. Today, I will be handing out individual spiral notebook journals to each of you to write in, and they will be for your eyes only unless, of course, you choose to share what you wrote in them with others. Okay? Let's get started."

I began passing out the journals. "I am passing out journals with your names on the front cover. These are yours to keep and write in. As you open them up, you will see several questions indexed 1-13, with each question including spaces to write in. We will begin working on the first of 13 questions tonight. Bring these journals to group from now on and to our individual counseling sessions. We will work on these together. Do you all understand what I am asking you to do?"

I checked in with each veteran in the group. Each nodded in agreement.

"Let me read to you the first questions in your journal. Remember, answering these questions may take some time and a lot of soul searching and deep consideration. So, there is no time limit to complete them, nor is there any requirement for the length of your notes. You can write pages or just paragraphs. This is for you. What you write, let it flow from your heart. Dig deep; don't hold back. It is private. It is yours."

I opened my journal and read the 13 questions aloud.

1. Have you seriously damaged your relationships with other people because of your negative attitudes and destructive behaviors? If so, list the relationships and how you damaged them.

2. If other people have told you how you have hurt them, write down what they said.

3. Describe times and ways that you have significantly neglected or damaged relationships with your loved ones because you were detaching or isolating.

4. Describe any physical damages that have resulted from your current behaviors.

5. Describe times that you have withdrawn from social interaction and activities and isolated yourself to an extreme degree and why.

6. Describe incidents where you expressed inappropriate anger towards other people.

7. Describe embarrassing or humiliating incidents in your life. Were they related to your war experiences or memories? If so, how were they related?

8. Describe attempts that you have made in the past to change or fix your out-of-control lifestyle. How successful have they been? Do these attempts show the powerlessness that you have over your damaging behaviors?

9. Do you feel any remorse from the ways that you have acted in your life? If so, explain that in detail.

10. Describe any irrational or crazy set of events that have happened since you came home from the war zones. Did you rationalize this behavior? If so, in what way?

11. Have you avoided people because they did not share in or approve of your lifestyle? If so, list these people and situations.

12. Can you pinpoint one time in your life when your life began to become extremely out of control? If so, describe that period and what was happening.

13. How would you summarize the powerlessness and unrestrained parts of your life in the face of your current behaviors?

After reading the questions, I asked the group, "Any of those questions trigger thoughts or considerations or concerns?"

I gave everyone a minute to think about it. There were no comments, so I continued, "There are huge benefits when you journal. You can use journaling to reduce stress, increase self-reflection, and create a better sense of wellbeing. One of the great things about journaling is there is no wrong way to do it. Journaling is all about dumping that stuff floating around in your head and then being able to walk away from it. By externalizing your thoughts and feelings through journaling, you may tend to have less to carry around psychologically. Your brain will thank you. Journaling also gives you the unique ability to look back and see how much you have grown, both emotionally and spiritually. Does that make sense to any of you?" A few of the vets nodded in agreement. I looked around the room. Alice Anderson raised her hand.

"Yes, Alice?" I acknowledged her as she leaned forward and sat upright in her chair.

"I have some questions. All these questions you just read to us, Vic…what if I can't find the words to express my true feelings or don't even want to answer the question?"

"Alice, I certainly can understand it if you must hesitate or have difficulty identifying sensitive emotions to write about. Some things may be difficult to express right now. Give it time. Keep it simple. One of the ways to deal with any overwhelming emotion is to find a healthy way to express yourself. This makes a journal a helpful tool in managing your mental health. Journaling can also help you manage your anxiety, cope with depression, and control your symptoms. Alice, you may find writing things down will improve your mood by helping you prioritize and identify problems, fears, and concerns. Tracking any symptoms day-to-day will help you recognize triggers and learn ways to better control them. Make any sense? Does that help you?"

Alice sat back in her chair, arms folded, and responded, "Some."

"Excellent," I said, turning to see if others in the circle wanted to talk.

Corporal Maxwell spoke up without raising his hand. "I have something to say."

He nervously shifted in his chair. His face was scarred in places near his hair line, and chewing-tobacco stains shadowed the corners of his mouth. He spoke in a low voice. "Those questions you want us to write about seem personal, Vic, a lot of relationship kinds of shit. How's that going to help me stop using drugs? I'm an addict, not an author." Some anxious vets in the group, chuckled.

"Good question, Jimmy. Let me answer your concern this way. Addiction involves craving for something intensely, loss of control over its use, and continuing involvement with it despite adverse behavior or consequences. Does that sound accurate?"

Corporal Maxwell just stared at me. I continued, "addiction changes the brain, first by disrupting the way it registers pleasure, and then by corrupting other normal drives such as learning and motivation. Someone with an addiction will crave a substance or display other obsessive habits. They'll often ignore other areas of life to fulfill or support their desires. General signs are lack of control or inability to stay away from the substance or behavior. Does that sound like someone you know, Mr. Maxwell?" Jimmy grinned slightly, rubbing his chin.

"So, Jimmy, keeping a journal helps you create order when your world feels like it's in chaos. You get to know yourself by revealing your most private fears, thoughts, and feelings, providing an opportunity for positive self-talk and identifying negative thoughts and behaviors. These are things we can work on privately in our one-on-one counseling sessions in my office or in group if you feel comfortable sharing with the others. My recommendation for all of you is to look at your writing time as personal relaxation time. It's a time when you can wind down and dig deep. Write in a place that's relaxing and soothing, maybe with a cup of coffee. Look forward to your journaling time. Know that you're doing something good for your mind, heart, and soul, and I will be there to help you every step of the way if you will let me." I was looking Jimmy squarely in the eyes. I saw a bit of moisture collecting around his eyelids. He looked away.

I continued engaging the rest of the group, saying, "When you have a problem and you're stressed, keeping a journal can help you identify what's causing that stress or anxiety. Once you've identified your stressors, we can work on your treatment action plan goals to resolve the problems and reduce your stress. Any questions or comments?"

The room fell silent.

"We will be wrapping up group in a few minutes. I have just one more important thing I would like to say to you tonight. Please, keep in mind that journaling is just one of many aspects of a balanced lifestyle we will be working on during the next 18 months."

I got up out of my chair and walked around the room to make sure everyone was on board and engaged. Then, I concluded the meeting with some final instructions and encouragement.

"Your healthy lifestyles should always include relaxation and meditation each day as well as eating a healthy, balanced diet. And exercise regularly—get in some activity every day even if it is just a walk around the block. And, listen-up—very important—treat yourself to plenty of sleep each night and obviously stay away from alcohol and drugs. I will be drug screening you randomly, so stay clean. Capisce? One final thing before you go: try these tips to help you get started writing in your journals. Set aside a few minutes every day to write. Keep it simple, Make it easy. Always keep a pen handy. Then, when you want to write down your thoughts, you can. You can also keep a journal in a computer file if that will be easier for you. Write whatever feels right. Your journal doesn't need to follow any certain structure. It's your own private place to discuss whatever you want. Let the words flow freely. Don't worry about spelling mistakes or what other people might think. Use your journal as you see fit.

You don't have to share your journal with anyone. If you do want to share some of your thoughts with me or the group or trusted friends and loved ones, you could show them all or part of it. That's it for tonight, everyone. Good work! I'm so proud of each one of you. Remember your individual appointment times with me this week, to work on your treatment plans, right? See you all later."

I opened the door and left the room.

# CHAPTER 2

# Abandonment

I have found time and time again working with veterans that what saves lives is developing a new sense of purpose, one built on a transformed and positive identity. For Sergeant Jake Storm, the absolute crucial part to that process was the act of gut-level storytelling while living in the present—acknowledging and laying to rest the actions of his past. Over time and after building trust, I began to identify the type of talk and storytelling that empowered Jake, guiding and encouraging him every step of the way.

I vividly remember the first day I met Sergeant Storm. He was slumped awkwardly in the waiting room chair, cautiously surveying the layout of the clinic, his back to the wall, as if casing the place. A camouflage utility cover tilted down over the right side of his furrowed forehead, partially covering his squinting blue eyes. Just by looking at his solid shoulders, muscular posture, and partially hidden face features, I felt I already knew a part of this warrior's story.

This was the beginning of weeks and months Jake Storm and I worked together on the principal cornerstone of utilizing my ability to sustain heart-to-heart responsiveness with him during our conversations in my private office and with the other veterans in Group Room #2. This was the exact time when and where the model of Heart-to-Heart Resuscitation began to take shape and become real.

In Sergeant Storm's mind, the sun had just broken through the early morning fog bank along the beach breakwater of the Marine Corps Base Camp Pendleton, California. The waves broke on the reef rocks in front of Jake, casting a fine mist onto his graying whiskered face. The brackish seawater mist joined the salt from the tears rolling down his cheeks. The tide was rolling in. As he gazed upon the scene, his furrowed facial features looking deep into the ocean water's sudsy edge, in his mind's eye he carefully observed the tide action in the ocean's surf. Always fascinated by the vastness of the ocean, the Vietnam Marine veteran stood with amazed admiration as he watched the tide effects on the ocean and its habitation. He closed his eyes, his face catching the breeze as clouds began to swallow his mind.

Jake Storm's thoughts continued to wander. He seemed constantly to be playing back tapes that spun on and on, disappearing into the mist. He visualized large, old-fashioned metal reels, spinning in a never-ending loop.

Jake's lessons began at an early age. Not pleasant at times. Jake's parents divorced when he was four years old. He couldn't remember being held or nurtured by his mother or father. No ball games with Dad. A small voice in his head often told him to suck it up and get over it. His room at home and in the military boarding school always seemed cold and empty, void of feeling. Something or someone was missing. The pain of abandonment dominated his soul. The tide was out most of the time in his early childhood, empty and shallow, forever retreating like the water's edge from the sand. He felt deformed and detached most of the time growing up. Whose child am I, anyway? He often reflected.

Jake had no early connectedness. His thoughts become distant when he tried to identify with connectedness between human beings. He remembered no attachments. The ocean scene returned to his mind. Do not the dolphin and her calf create a secure bond, improving the calf's chances for survival? He deliberated. Reflecting on the notion, he accepted the wisdom the baby instinctually knows the caregiver is dependable, which seems to create a secure base for the calf then to explore. This baby calf knows its parent will provide comfort and reassurance, so is comfortable seeking it out in times of need. As the seasoned Vietnam vet looked off into the vastness of the blue skies, he thought about how this in-the-wild relationship evoked the strength of nature. The former Marine scuba diver imagined the baby dolphin, swimming close to its mother and carried in the mother's slip stream, the hydrodynamic wake that develops as the mother swims. Did I ever have a dynamic wake to guide me as a child? He thought about this question in a distant, deeply abstract way.

Jake's initial voyage of discovery and emotional development began as a big disappointment. Maternal deprivation came to mind as he watched the seagulls soaring above him. How nicely the birds flocked as a family, gliding together up and down and around each other and landing on the soft sandy beach head in groups, he thought to himself. There was something warm and peaceful about this image. Inspired for the moment, he managed a smile. In fact, he began to speak bird-talk to the swarming seagulls as if they could understand his gibberish. On occasion, Jake would bring a bag full of breadcrumbs down to the beach and feed the seagulls out of his hand. He liked the rare natural moments of feeding birds in the wild. Jake would not go to the zoo. He despised people who caged any form of wildlife.

Caught in layers of memories, Jake's mind moved to another moment of his past. He had remained in country when he and several of his buddies were honorably discharged from the service. Most were decorated combat veterans. The term, *in country*, in this case referred not to the jungles of Vietnam anymore but to the hills and mountain ranges of the Sierra Nevada. Sarge walked out of the El Toro Marine Corps Air Station in California a free man—and an angry veteran. The day he and his friends left the main gate of the base, they were greeted by anti-war protestors chanting and holding signs with negative propaganda and demeaning slogans like "U.S. Imperialism" and "Get out of Vietnam." This was about the time that 20,000-30,000 people staged the huge "Human Be-In" anti-war event that took place in Golden Gate Park, San Francisco in early 1967. The discharged Marines were told about possible protestors but never expected such a negative homecoming. Sarge and his Marine Corps buddies felt abandoned. The men were outraged and demoralized and wanted nothing to do with civilians, so they set up a survival tent camp, sheltered by camouflage fabric, located at the North Fork of the Kings River about 100 miles east of Fresno, California. They moved there and lived off the land for several years.

Jake sat, alone, hair and beard showing signs of gray, enveloped in self-indulgent self-pity. As he scanned the distant horizon for fishing boats, his imagination traveled without destination. He found himself wiping the tears intermittently undulating down his face from his slightly swollen, wrinkled eye sockets, thinking about life gone by.

As Jake watched the seagulls play in the sky, the salty sea mist cooled his face. A memory came to mind. He always enjoyed the moment when Grandpa would ask his awkward, young grandson to assist him in putting on his wooden leg. When his parents were in the throes of working out a divorce in the early years of his life, Jake lived with his grandparents quite often. These things he did not understand, of course, at the age of innocence.

Jake recalls putting on the large, soft, cotton stocking that covered his grandfather's stump. Then, Jake would go over to the chair beside his bed and carry the shiny, polished, wooden leg to him. He would help him slip it on and strap it to his thigh and waist. Then, he would go over to the dresser drawer that he knew so well and pick out a set of socks for him to wear that day. He would put the socks on his grandpa's feet—both the wooden foot and the natural one. Grandpa would pat his grandson on the head and smile. Jake felt his love even though he couldn't remember his grandfather ever telling him he loved him. Jake just knew it.

The whirlpools down the slope in front of Jake swirled among the rocky reef as if for a moment the marine life was caught up in a washing machine spin cycle. As Jake approached the tidal waters on the rocky shore, a hermit crab scampered across the light-brown sand between the rocks, seeking shelter under crusty stones covered with small marine invertebrate animals enclosed in spherical shells. Jake carefully kneeled down to join their world. Kneeling in the salty, foamy sea water, he couldn't help but notice the beautiful colors emanating from the reef rocks around him. Purple spine sea urchins clustered about the stones and rocks. There must be hundreds of them. He gently put his rather large, thick finger in the center of one of them. The soft, slimy, spherical sea animal welcomed Jake into its world with a soft squeeze, closing in on his index finger. He grinned, feeling a simple pleasure of life that provided a moment of relief.

Jake settled in, his muscular knees sinking into the wet swirling sand, With the keen sense of a sniper's eye, he observed the sea creature's world as well as other interesting wildlife floating about in their busy little space. Jake's swirling memory took him back in time. Not all was a happy little space in Jake's world. In his early years and beyond, he remembered the loneliness he felt as a child growing up. He wondered how a wounded dolphin might feel, sensing it is vulnerable to predators on the hunt at any moment. Or how an aging tortoise feels, swirling stiff and slow, caught up in the surf, and coming to shore for rest in a weak position and exposed.

Jake was always troubled by those small voices in his head. The doctors at the Naval Hospital at Camp Pendleton Marine Base suggested that he suffered from post-traumatic stress disorder (PTSD). At times, Sarge felt that he did have emotional and personal problems. He thought about his difficulties controlling his emotions and poor social skills. He couldn't keep a job—he had had many. He often wondered about his persistent sadness and negative thoughts, including disturbing thoughts about suicide.

No counseling or therapy was mandated at the time when Jake returned home from the war in Vietnam. He felt isolated most of the time. For years, he had been experiencing altercations in relations with others; he trusted almost no one. Sudden, loud noises—any number of things other people don't even notice—acted as a trigger back to his intense war experiences.

Nam took a lot out of this giant of a man. He was barely 20 years old when his Marine Company first arrived on the beachhead of Red Beach in Vietnam in 1965. He and his Marine buddies were told their sole purpose was to provide protection to the American air base at Danang. In fact, the official directive was: "The U.S. Marine force will not engage in day-to-day actions against the Viet Cong." However, as the U. S. expanded its build-up with additional bases south at Chu Lai and north at Phu Bai, these rules of limited engagement became increasingly difficult to maintain. Jake was a combat Marine. Rated "expert" on the range in Camp Matthews, he was a "grunt" riflemen, trained to kill. He wanted and waited to use his keenly honed skills, spending hours cleaning and maintaining his battle equipment, using a finely grained sedimentary rock as a whetstone for sharpening razors and other cutting tools. He favored his 11-inch, black carbon USMC Fighting Knife, which he had strapped to his leg bindings in its leather sheath. Jake was so proficient with this weapon he could throw and hit a marker on a tree 20 feet away.

The Viet Cong set up strongholds in neighboring villages from where they would launch attacks against Jake and his search-and-destroy unit. His command soon recognized that in order to protect the American bases, these pockets of resistance needed to be flushed out. The South Vietnamese Army (RVN) had responsibility for securing the countryside, but it was soon apparent they were not able to do so without assistance from the American forces. Jake's company commander received word that the initial directive was expanded to allow Marines to work with the RVN soldiers in areas critical to U. S. security. Jake and his buddies knew that that meant action was coming.

In the Vietnam War, intelligence was never precise, and Jake's company had landed right in the middle of the Vietcong 60th Battalion and found itself surrounded. The VC let the first helicopters land without incident, then opened on succeeding waves, a tactic they had used successfully against the South Vietnamese's Army. Three U.S. Army UH-lB helicopter gunships were called in to strafe the VC stronghold, a small knoll called Hill 34. Meanwhile, Jake's patrol teams protected the landing zones until the full company had landed. The company commander ordered an assault on the hill by one platoon, but it quickly stalled.

Regrouping his men, his platoon leader realized that he had happened upon a heavy concentration of Vietcong. The Captain ordered in strikes against Hill 34 and then assaulted it with all three of his platoons. Reinforced by close air support, Jake's rifle squads overran the enemy position, claiming six VC killed in action at one machine-gun position alone. Hill 34 was taken. It was here Jake received his first experience of how to kill. He was awarded a field promotion to the rank of Sergeant E-5. And so, Jake's combat legacy began.

As Jake focused on life in the tide pool, he realized the red reef hermit crab had floated against his leg, testing his skin softly with fire engine red pinchers. He began to wonder what she could be thinking. She was beautiful and feminine, gliding in the surf, looking up at him with protruding yellow eyestalks. As he continued watching, the hermit crab retreated to her cave. He reached out to gently touch her shell. Watching her in action encouraged Jake's thinking, when am I going to stop running and come out of hiding?

Suddenly, the muscles in his stomach tightened. His teeth began to clench, and his throat ached. He had to restrain himself from bellowing out sensitive feelings that were burning to escape, the pain of so many years.

Jake had a major battle going on inside. His mind was reeling; he felt friendless and alone in the battle. Who could care enough to really understand him? If he killed himself, no one would miss him. It would end his pain. His mind spun like the current in the tide pool. How could he ever forget the devastating agony and helplessness he felt the day his Marine buddy was killed by a sniper's bullet, blood gurgling out of his neck and down his face from his nose—Jake's first smell of blood, the touch of hot fluid running through Jake's fingers as he tried to stop the blood flow from the wound.

Jake was so young in battle, so confused, and alone. His body filled with fear—and anger and rage. The tears began to run, dripping off his nose into the tide pool. Sergeant Jake Storm was a volcano about to erupt.

Jake found himself sinking into the sandy beach around the rocks. His head was drenched in salt water he gasped for air and rose up from the outgoing tide, exclaiming, "I am a coward!" Thoughts raced through his head. He was still alive, not having allowed the retreating tide to carry him out to sea to freedom's welcoming arms. Where were his Marine buddies? Why was it not he who took the sniper's bullets that pierced his best friend's neck? Guilt permeated his heart and soul. "I have no need to live another day. Oh, God take me!" he screamed out as the echo of his words jumped between the rolling waves. He paused, looking out over the ocean, wiping his eyes with the backs of his huge, aging hands, and squinting into the sunlight's glaring rays and stinging reflection from the Pacific Ocean edge. Then, he stood up, turned quickly to look over his shoulder as if he was startled by a noise, and moved quickly down the beach.

Jake had long experienced periods of mental disturbances, abnormal behavior, and recurring PTSD symptoms. He was told that his war traumas caused his behavior, and he believed it to be so. So often he found himself wrestling with flashbacks that contained a mixture of real and imaginary characters, places, and events.

Some years back, he began drinking heavily. Whiskey helped him sleep. He was warned about mixing some of his medications with booz, but he did it, anyway. One day in September, he drank until passing out.

Jake continued walking down the sloping, soft sand, still a bit unsettled by his thoughts. He hesitated for a moment, crouched down, and lunged toward an elongated stem-like structure. Aggressively, he began stomping on the gas-filled bladders of sea kelp. Under the weight of his huge feet the bladders popped like gun shots. This seemed to amuse Jake. He managed a smile. He knew from instinct the enemy was close at hand. He began to run, sprinting wildly, yelling at the top of his lungs until his throat burned.

When he finally stopped, he fell forward on his knees, arms outstretched and beefy hands clutching at the sand. He began to sob. He lowered his head lowered in anguish. His face settled into the sand, the powerful current of his hot breath blowing a hollow cavity under his opened mouth into the sand; his teeth bit into the shores' coarse granules.

After some moments, he heard foreign voices approaching. He began hearing all-too-familiar attack screams. He tilted his head again, cocking his ear in the direction of the sounds. In slow motion, familiar Viet Cong faces began to pop out of the fog bank. One appeared from the right flank, another from the left, coming right at him, firing an AK 47. Jake ducked, desperately searching for his weapon and for cover. He tried frantically to stand up and defend himself. He looked for his buddies for back up. He was alone.

Jake awoke at home mid-afternoon, dripping wet with perspiration, his body shaking. He found himself crouching on all fours under the top sheet and blanket of his bed covers. Suddenly, he felt suffocated, trapped, held down by the weight of the covers. He panicked, tearing at the sheet, and then, losing his balance, he rolled off the bed, covers and all, hitting the wood paneled floor.

For a moment, Jake lost all sense of where he was. He labored to breath. After a few moments, he rolled onto his side and began looking around his small apartment. He shook his head trying to make sense out of what he had just experienced. That same nightmare, again and again, he thought. "Just too real, too much to take, I'm tired," he muttered to himself, shaking his head again and again as if that would release the nightmarish dream. Still on his side, leaning limply on his right elbow, his head partly raised, Jake began scanning the apartment as if seeking something familiar.

His eyes suddenly focused in on his side table, next to the bed. Anxiously, he began pushing and kicking the covers off his naked legs. He scooted himself across the lacquer floorboards, then reached up and opened the table drawer. He extended his long arm into the drawer, shuffling around with his hand. He paused; his arm action stopped as he found what he had been seeking.

He gripped cold metal and pulled from the drawer from the side table drawer a semi-automatic pistol, the standard-issue side arm for the United States Armed Forces. Oh, he knew it well! In fact, he could tear it down and reassemble it blindfolded in under a minute. In Vietnam, ,,he wore it as a sidearm every day, even when he was sleeping. During the war, he had carried it cradled in a linseed-oiled, cowhide-leather shoulder holster under his left arm. That weapon had saved his life and lives of others during several firefights and close combat encounter on Hill 34.

Jake was still sitting on the floor, leaning against his bed. He stared at the weapon resting in his lap. The custom leather wrapped pistol grip was indenting his thigh, the barrel pointing between his bare legs. Once again, tears splashed against his chiseled cheek bones and rapelled down his beard. He tightened his grip on his weapon until his hand turned white, bloodless, throbbing from emotion. Then, with blurry eyes, he looked down and pushed the clip release on his weapon, dropping the clip into his hand and intently studied it.

Seven rounds, he contemplated as if taking a quick ammo count before a firefight: standard-capacity magazine, muzzle velocity 800 feet per second, effective range 75 yards on a good day. Today is a good day to die, he thought.

As he raised the full clip in front of his face, he studied the single protruding round—a torpedo ready for launch. He quickly jammed the magazine clip back into the pistol handle, pulling back the slide and sending the bullet into the chamber, while cocking the weapon and releasing the safety all in a 2-second motion.

Tired and confused, he slowly closed his eyes and rested his head against the bed mattress for several minutes. Methodically, Jake he lifted the pistol toward his head. Tears trickled. He pushed the barrel up under his chin as his index finger danced around the trigger grazing it oh, so slightly. The weapon was in place. He breathed rapidly, and his hand quivered.

Time passed, and then, suddenly, he relaxed, lowering the side arm to the floor, still loaded and ready to fire. He exhaled and yelled out, "If there is a God, I need you now… not tomorrow, not next year…right now, God!" Jake dropped his head between his elevated knees and began to cry feverishly.

In his initial days of PTSD diagnosis and treatment, Jake had received many hours of therapy and group counseling for survivor's guilt as well as flashbacks and the nightmares he experienced. Several times in treatment he was asked about suicide ideation. At the time he felt immune to the possibility of taking his own life. But years had passed.

Jake, still leaning on the sink basin in front of the mirror, heard a hard-knuckle knock on the apartment's wooden door. The noise startled Jake who rarely had visitors at this hou—or at any time, for that matter. He quickly shuffled across the bedroom as if guarding a dribbling basketball player and then crouched to look around the corner and between the slightly opened bedroom door toward the front door, his loaded-and-cocked weapon in his right hand. He waited.

A familiar voice accompanied a second knock. "Sarge, Sarge, it's Corporal Rodriquez. I am in your men's group at the vet center. Remember, I fought with you in Nam."

An eerie silence filled the air. Jake continued to glare hypnotically at the front door, as if he could see through it. "Sarge," the corporal continued, "I haven't seen you in group for weeks, I came over tonight to see if you are alright."

Jake moved cautiously toward the front door raising his weapon behind his back with his right hand tucking the barrel of the .45 into the waistband of his skivvies. He put his head against the door, "Rodriquez, what's up?"

"Sarge, may I come in for a minute? I have something I want to give you."

With his left hand, Jake slowly opened the door. The corporal was standing in the hallway and held what appeared to be an envelope in his hand.

"Hey, Sarge, Semper Fi! I received this letter in the mail from Veteran Affairs last week and thought you may want to look at it."

Jake looked down at the envelope in the corporal's hand and took it, giving Rodriquez an empty stare.

"I have your back, Sarge. I owe you my life. Oorah!"

As the corporal walked away, Jake managed under his breath, "Oorah, Rodriquez, Semper Fi!"

The corporal heard his sergeant's words but never turned around. Tears welled as he walked away down the hall.

Jake closed the door and pounded his forehead into the back of it several times, then used his balled fist. He was at a crossroads and exhausted. He flopped down on the closest chair, stared at the loaded pistol for a couple of minutes, and then set it on the table next to the chair. The white envelope rested on his lap. Tired of fighting his demons, he closed his eyes and fell asleep.

The next morning, Jake opened the envelope. Still slumping in his chair, Jake began to read the one-page letter inside:

Department of Veteran Affairs
Under Secretary for Health
Washington, DC 20420

Dear Veteran,

If you're experiencing an emotional crisis and need to talk with a trained VA professional, the National Suicide Prevention Hotline toll-free number, 1-800-273-TALK (8255), is now available 24 hours a day, 7 days a week. You will immediately be connected with a qualified and caring provider who can help.

Here are some suicide warning signs:

1. Threatening to hurt or kill yourself
2. Looking for ways to kill yourself
3. Seeking access to pills, weapons, and other self-destructive behavior
4. Talking about death, dying or suicide

The presence of these signs requires immediate attention. If you or a veteran you care about has been showing any of these signs, do not hesitate to call and ask for help!

Additional warning signs may include:

1. Hopelessness
2. Rage, anger, seeking revenge
3. Acting reckless or engaging in risky activities, seemingly without thinking
4. Increasing alcohol or drug abuse
5. Feeling trapped- like there's no way out
6. Withdrawing from friends and family
7. Anxiety, agitation, inability to sleep- or excessive sleepiness
8. Dramatic mood swings
9. Feeling there's no reason for living, no sense of purpose in life

Please call the toll-free hotline number, 1-800-273- TALK (8255) if you experience any of these warning signs. We'll get you the help and assistance you need right away!

Sincerely yours,
Michael J. Kussman, MD, MS, MACP

Jake's eyes scanned the letter quickly top to bottom. What is Rodriquez thinking? Why is he giving me this letter? Returning thoughtfully to the beginn[ing of the letter, he began to read it out loud to himself, hesitating at several points. When he had finished, he let the paper drop onto his lap. Jake clenched his teeth at the message he was getting loud and clear. Get help, Sergeant Storm, get help—now, before it is too late.

A month earlier, Jake's youngest sister, Samantha, his favorite sibling (of three sisters and a half-brother) and the only one who kept in constant contact with him over the years, had come by to check up on her big brother. She visited from time to time, inviting him to church and wanting to talk about their good childhood memories and the Bible. She would leave spiritual tracks and booklets for him to read, like the *Our Daily Bread* devotional. He never could bring himself to open them up. He would throw them into the bottom drawer of his dresser.

Jake recalled her saying, "I am not talking about religious doctrines or affiliations, Jake. I am talking about a personal relationship. There is a huge difference. There is hope and healing in Jesus." Jake never really understood what she meant by a personal relationship with Jesus, but he knew she meant well and so shrugged it off.

Jake rejected the notion of religion. Oh, he would always say he believed in God. Certainly, most combat warriors he served with, including himself, had foxhole religion when the heat was on in a firefight or incoming motor rounds were blazing and shells exploding, sending hot chucks of steel everywhere around them. But for Sarge, and so many other seasoned combat veterans, believing in something unseen, something or someone they can't touch or hear is difficult. They are survivors of the killing fields. Most had to rely on their own skills and strength to get through the bloody battles. For many, anything spiritual was a foreign thought.

Indeed, Jake was stuck. Spiritually he felt empty although on two Sundayshe had slipped into the back pew in a church down the street, hoping not to be noticed. Psychologically he wasn't able to function without help from anti-depressants and doctors. Alcohol became his God.

Jake picked up the Veteran Affairs letter and studied it. He read the words, "if you're experiencing an emotional crisis and need to talk," over and over. His eyes zeroed in on sentences "threatening to hurt or kill yourself and looking for ways to kill yourself" and "seeking access to weapons and other self-destructive behavior." The words, "the presence of these signs requires immediate attention," jumped off the page. For a brief moment, he studied his load .45 still sitting on the end table.

Jake had never really opened up and shared his true feelings with anyone in all the years he attended veteran groups and therapy. He felt safer keeping the emotions to himself. He also did not believe in shrinks. Not even nice ones. He went to therapy only to receive his sleeping pills and pain relievers. And because he promised his sister that he would keep going.

Jake contemplated the words, "hopelessness...feeling trapped... withdrawing from friends and family...feeling there is no reason for living, no sense of purpose in life." He squinted in deep thought.

Today happened to be Sunday. Jake lifted himself out of the chair and walked over to the window. Leaning forward to get a better look down the street, he saw people gathering in front of the church. He turned to the clock on the wall: 8:37. The church bells would be ringing at 9:00.

There was something very different about this Sunday morning. As Jake approached the church, he felt unsettled. His heart ached; his stomach twisted. He had arrived just in time for the bells. Proceeding to the rear of the church, he picked out a pew bench that looked safe; his back would be to the outer wall. He felt safer sitting that way when in public places.

The church began to fill up. Jake had wished many times he could tell a minister about his pain but was afraid.

As he waited for the opening hymn, he began looking high above the altar. A very large white cross hung diagonally from the ceiling. Beautiful, he thought. As he stared up at the cross, the organist began to play. His eyes uncontrollably filled with tears. What is going on here? In the past, he had had a comfortable feeling when entering the doors of this church. So, what was the big deal now?

The church for Jake served as a sanctuary away from the madding crowds of people and fast-paced society that tore at his soul. The pressures and troubles of his world faded away while he sat there, leaving him with a rarely experienced sense of peace.

As the choir sang. Jake looked around, carefully and guarded, so no one could see the tears he was fighting back. The hymns were upbeat full of praise and worship. With blurred vision, he looked for anyone else with teary eyes. No one. So, why was he crying?

Suddenly, his stomach muscles tensed, and his teeth clenched. He had to restrain himself from shouting out. The years of suppressed pain were overwhelming. A battle raged inside him. What was happening to him? He could not remember ever feeling this torn up, alone in battle, abandoned. Who could care enough to really understand him? Men had died on his watch in Vietnam. How was he to live with that? Who cared about the abandonment and rejection he felt as a child or the abuse, and the cruelty of being separated and sent away from his family when he was 7 years old, fatherless? Who could possibly forgive an alcoholic who used and abused many people for many years? How could he ever forget the devastating pain and helplessness he felt the day the sheriff came and took Jake's boys away because he was too drunk and out of control to be allowed to be their father? Who could love or forgive such a man?

For a moment, Jake considered running out of the church as the pastor was preaching his sermon. He barely heard the message. He was crying out from his insides, "Oh, God, help me! I need you."

The sermon seemed to last forever. Jake was waiting for something to happen. He needed something to happen. The letter he was given by Corporal Rodriquez had convinced him that he needed help. And he needed help from God.

The pastor invited to the altar those who wanted God in their lives, His forgiveness, and eternal salvation. This was the moment his little sis had been talking about. This must be it. The sign from God. He could feel it, but he hesitated. No one had come forward. A million thoughts raced through Jake's confused brain. What would everyone think about him? Look at that big combat-hardened Marine vet, devil dog, leatherneck, macho man on his knees at the altar, crying like a baby? Time passed. Jake's feet would not move. He began leaning in the direction of the aisle, hoping his feet would follow to the altar. They did not. He felt numb all over. The Sarge who fought so many firefights and had so many kills could not move an inch. He was frozen in place. Tears streamed down his cheeks.

Church was over. Jake quickly wiped his eyes on his shirt sleeves, but as he slowly moved out of the main sanctuary into the foyer, his tears returned. He turned on his heel to escape attention and hurried toward a small doorway 20 feet away.

As he touched the door handle, a volcano began to erupt from deep within his body and soul. He opened the door, not knowing what to expect. and quickly shut it behind him. No one was there. He had entered a prayer chapel.

Dimly lit, the chapel had a dozen wooden pews and a short aisle to the modest altar. The cross on the wall seemed larger than life and beamed with a radiance that Jake would never forget. His eyes swollen with tears and his legs weak, he could not move even the short distance to the altar. He fell to the floor on his knees and crawled the rest of the way.

Driven to his knees in front of the radiant cross, Jake cried out, "God forgive me. Please forgive me! Oh, God, forgive me! I need you in my life. I am a killer of men, not worthy to live another day." He began rocking back and forth on his knees. Tears and the prayers for help continued to spew forth. Emotionally spent, Jake sensed something different around him: a quiet calm he cannot explain even to this day.

Jake fell silent. The only noise in the room was his occasional exhausted sigh. he remained on his knees for what seemed a lifetime.

Jake tried to get up, but nothing worked. His legs had no strength. He reached over to the nearest pew and pulled himself up onto the seat, where he rested for a moment. An unspeakable burden had been removed.

Returning to his apartment, Jake glanced down the hallway as if looking for Corporal Rodriquez and recalled the last words the corporal had said to him, "I have your back, Sarge."

Once home and settled, Jake opened the frig. Not much in there. He must get to the market. He pulled out a half-used package of lunch meat and threw it on the table. A loaf of white bread was sitting in the corner cabinet. Normally, Jake was a big eater but not in recent weeks. He found eating interfered with his drinking. Jake sat down at the table and threw together a bologna sandwich. As he began to chow down his first meal in several days, he thought about his sister Sam. She would have wanted to be with me this morning. I owe her my life.

He finished the sandwich and then retrieved the letter from the VA. As he picked it up from the table, he bumped the custom grip of the .45 spinning it around. He noticed the hammer remained back and ready to fire. The safety was off. Jake reached for the weapon. He carefully uncocked the hammer with his right thumb and put the safety in place. Then, he walked into his bedroom and opened the side-table drawer and placed the weapon back where he normally kept it.

Back at the kitchen table, he re-read the letter from the Veteran Affairs Department several times, always stopping at the hotline toll-free number. He was curious now. How could they help him? He was already on meds and saw a VA doc for 5 minutes every other month. What more could he need?

Suddenly serious, he realized that he did have many of the warning signs laid out in the letter. Who walks around with a loaded gun to their head, drinking themself to death? Oh, no, Sarge, you don't have a problem!

Jake stared at the phone hanging loosely on the wall. He just sat there and stared at it for what seemed the longest time. Then, feeling somewhat renewed with lifted spirits from his chapel experience in church, he made the call: 1-800-273-TALK. The phone rang at the other end. Jake suddenly felt some fear. What will I say? How can I trust this person I have never seen?

"Hello, you have reached the National Veterans Suicide Crisis Hotline,. My name is Al Stuart. How may I help you today?... Hello...Hello..."

Jake hit the switch and disconnected the call. "Shit!" he said shaking his head radically left and right. He put his head in his hands, elbows on the table. "Shit, shit, shit!" How tough was this? Well, Sergeant, you can't shoot yourself...now you can't even make a phone call... pathetic! And you call yourself a warrior. Get real! F___me!

Jake settled down in the next minutes, walked into the bathroom to take a wiz, then flopped down on a chair in the living room and switched on the television with a remote, flipping through the channels, looking at them with a blank stare. He turned it off.

"I can do this," he said. "I can do it for Sam... hell for me."

Jake made the call again, 1-800-273-TALK...ringing. What if it's the same guy, Al whatever his name was?

"Hello, you have reached the National Veterans Suicide Crisis Hotline. My name is Kelly   Petersen. How may I help you?"

"Hello." Jake began to speak. "I am a disabled Vietnam vet."

"What is your first name?" Kelly asked.

"Why do you need to know that?" Jake responded somewhat agitatedly.

"Because I told you mine. Isn't that fair?"

"Jake is my name."

"Well, Jake, how may I help you today?"

"I don't know exactly. I am thinking some strange things the last few days. I have nightmares… can't sleep much" Jake shared.

"Are you thinking about suicide?" the hotliner responded.

"I was last night," Jake answered.

"Have you done anything to hurt yourself today?" Kelly replied.

"No!" Jake said emphatically.

"What has changed since last night?" Kelly asked inquisitively.

"Church" Jake replied. "I went to church this morning."

"Will you tell me about church, Jake? What happened at church this morning?"

"I had a good conversation with God; that is what happened." Jake replied.

"How are you feeling right now? Are you drinking alcohol or taking any other drugs?" Kelly inquired cautiously.

"No booze today. As for the pills, just taking my antidepressants and anxiety pills that doesn't seem to work anymore. That's for my PTSD stuff." Jake replied.

"Do you have a gun?" Kelly asked.

"Yes."

"Where is the gun right now, Jake?"

"In my bedroom side-table drawer."

"Where are the bullets kept?"

"In the clip of my .45, which is in my weapon."

"Have you ever attempted suicide?"

"No, but I think about giving up. Last night, I almost did it. I have no reason for living. I have nothing to live for. I am just a burden to society and my sis.

She worries about me, I know. She always has. She is the most important person in my life. If I am not around, she won't have to worry about her big brother."

"Jake, is there anyway someone can come over and take your gun somewhere else, out of your hands just for a while until I can get you some help—a neighbor or relative, perhaps?" Kelly asked.

"No, just my sister, but she lives an hour away. I wouldn't want to involve her in this. She has a family. She would really be sick with worry if she knew about this. I can't do that to her." Jake replied.

"Our conversations and records are all very private and confidential. Your sister won't be involved unless you want her to be." Kelly said. "But you would kill yourself! You don't think that would devastate your sister, Jake?" Kelly was getting a little testy. Jake became silent. Kelly backed off.

"Tell me more about your suicide thoughts, Jake. What's been happening in your life to make you feel this way?" Kelly asked.

"I'm just tired of living. I have trouble sleeping. I have nightmares and flashbacks about things that happened decades ago in the Nam. The only way I can get to sleep is by filling up with pills and booze. I have a VA psych doc, but he only has time to see me every other month and then for just a few minutes. He gives me more pills or ups the dosage and sends me home. I'm not blaming him. He is a nice guy. All the docs over the years have been the same. They are medical doctors who hand out pills. Psychiatrists... What the hell do they know about the stink of body decay and death and emotional pain of watching a buddy die in my arms? But for all the years I have been coming to the VA for so called treatment, nobody seems to really care—I mean really care about what happens to me. Back in the '60s and '70s and even '80s, we Vietnam vets got the short end of the stick. Today, we old guys get stuck in a group with a bunch of younger vets, and everyone talks about their war stories. I am sick of war stories... sick of it!"

"Tell me more about the men's groups you have been in lately, Jake."

"You want to hear it, Kelly? Really hear it?" Jake's voice elevated.

"Yes." Kelly responded. "But Jake, we can talk about it only with the understanding that you don't get all worked up and upset. Slow down, and just talk to me; don't yell. I am trying to understand how I can get you the help you need right now. Okay, Jake? Just talk to me."

"Kelly, I don't need to hear about those sand niggers in Iraq or Afghanistan. I have my own stories and memories about Victor Charlie and the gooks of Vietnam. Hell, I was killing gooks before some of those guys were born. How about someone helping me get rid of some of these demons I carry around with me day in and day out. That's what is driving me up a wall. I can't stop the damn dreams and flashbacks—lit-up faces and lifeless eyes. That's just the beginning, Kelly."

"Jake, where are you living right now?"

"You mean my address?" Jake felt annoyed.

"No, Jake, What is your living situation? Do you have money to have a place to live?"

"Yes, I am on 100% disability. Not much money but enough to keep me off the streets, for now, anyway."

"Jake, I want to get you some help today, right now. I can have you transported to a safe environment in ten minutes if you will give me some information like your address and phone number and date of birth. Can you do that?"

"No way, Kelly! I can get around on my own. No EMTs for me. Thanks, but no thanks. I'm okay today. The gun is in the drawer, I'm not going to kill myself. I am feeling much better after church this morning. I just called to talk to someone and find out what this suicide crisis hotline was all about. A buddy gave me this letter saying to call the hotline if I need help. Well, I need help but not an ambulance." Jake said insistently.

"Okay, Jake. I am very glad to hear you are feeling better. But I would like to refer you to our Suicide Crisis Prevention Coordinator, Bill Elliott, a VA Medical Center Psychologist. He is a specialist in war trauma and PTSD treatment planning. I can arrange for him to contact you if you will give me your phone number and address. He can make arrangement with you to come by your place for a visit and talk with you about some of your concerns. Can we do that?"

"That sounds all right, Kelly. I will agree to do that…but no ambulance."

"No ambulance, I promise, Jake. Now, I need your address, phone number, and date of birth, and I will have Dr. Elliott get in touch with you in 24 hours or less. Sound good?"

"That's alright. Thanks for your help, Kelly. Here is that information." Jake responded.

"Jake, please always remember, if you ever need help and support in the future, don't hesitate to call us again, any time 24/7. We are here for you. Welcome home!"

The next day Jake connected with Bill Elliott of the Crisis Prevention Coordinators team at the Veteran Medical Center located about 10 miles from where he was living. At this critical point on his lengthy path to recovery, he was referred to me for a complete current mental health evaluation, psychosocial assessment, suicide screening, and the development of treatment plan goals and objectives. His story conveys the perseverance he needed to get help even if it has been a long time coming.

By the time I had first met Sergeant Jake Storm at my outpatient clinic, he had already been diagnosed and treated for Vietnam combat fatigue after his discharge from the United States Marine Corps in 1970. After years of Cognitive Processing Therapy at the VA, which involved educating Jake about PTSD symptoms and cognitive changes in the areas of safety and trust, he continued to struggle. PTSD had not yet been defined or considered for coding in the Diagnostic and Statistical Manual of Mental Disorders (DSM- II). Ultimately, the American Psychological Association accepted the term, *post-traumatic stress disorder*, and the new diagnosis criterion became the classification for combat fatigue and was published as PTSD in the DSM-III in 1980.

Despite the enormous psychological toll Vietnam took on Jake's life, he had received far from a "hero's welcome" when he returned to the United States. He faced homecoming alone, alongside a few buddies who had shared their experiences but could offer only limited psychological support. When Jake arrived in the U.S., he was not applauded for his sacrifice but was often met with hostile demonstrations by anti-war activists. American society offered little acceptance of Vietnam veterans even years after the war. Many warriors returning home from the field of combat had a form of battle neurosis which was mostly seen in soldiers nearing the end of their tours and would likely have long-term consequences.

Imagine for a moment, you are 20 years old, a recruit grunt plodding in the middle of the night through a foreign angry jungle 8,500 miles from home. Picture yourself trudging along in this hostile country with every inch of your rucksack and fatigues drenched with a heavy dampness, vigilantly listening and squinting on high alert for any threatening sound or movement in the dark and always remembering what the drill instructors in boot camp had told you about the fate of the warriors who stepped on a trip-wire, setting off explosives, or fell into a hidden pit of bamboo sharpened punji sticks.

This honorable and courageous man is not unlike many other combat veterans returning home today from the deserts of Iraq and Afghanistan and other hot spots around the world. Wherever the war or conflict is fought, be it in the sandy arid deserts, jungles and mangrove swamps of Vietnam, the mountains, forests and woodlands of Korea, or the amphibious landings on the islands of the Pacific; it does not change the enormity of the human cruelty and tragic events seen and experienced that lie beyond many veteran's abilities to cope.

The presenting symptoms of Sergeant Storm's Vietnam combat fatigue included insomnia and recurrent terrifying nightmares. He constantly experienced reliving the severe psychic trauma of friends and fellow combatants being severely injured, mutilated, or killed. Guilt constantly distressed Sergeant Storm. Days of depression haunted him; Guilt over not having saved his buddy's life tormented him.

It was at this point I began to talk to him about how his traumatic war experiences mixed with his early childhood environment had deeply affected his mind, heart, and soul. I introduced the Model of Heart-to-Heart Resuscitation of motivational interviewing and person-centered unconditional positive regard counseling which differs sharply from the psychodynamic and behavioral approaches. The Affective Client Centered approach suggests that Jake would be better helped if he were encouraged to focus on his current subjective understanding rather than on some unconscious motive or someone else's interpretation of his situation. And until Sergeant Storm was able to reach out and trust someone while exploring the deepest levels of his innermost self— allowing himself to grieve properly and to tell his story—he would continue to suffer.

Successful recovery finally came with the rebuilding of a useful and positive identity. This was challenging, as the solution then was dependent on his willingness to participate, but we can all help our veterans get there by realizing we can relate to them as human beings.

After 20 months, I finally was able to balance Jake's Care Plan by providing him with new skills to manage his painful emotions and suicidal thoughts. Jake and I were specifically focused on healing skills.

1. The first skill was being deliberate, actively attentive, and focusing on improving his ability to accept and be present in the current moment. I introduced Jake to journaling to express himself.

2. Second, it was obvious he needed to learn about distress tolerance geared toward increasing his acceptance of negative emotion, rather than trying to escape from it or end his life.

3. Third, and a huge step in his treatment plan commitment, we role-played his emotion regulation, covering strategies to manage and change intense emotions that were causing many of his problems.

4. Fourth, I also worked with Jake on his interpersonal effectiveness skills consisting of strategies related to conflict resolution and effective communication that allowed him to communicate with others in a way that was assertive but maintained self-respect and strengthened relationships—family relationships, to start.

Today, Jake is reunited with his family. He has discovered he is a grandfather. Jake spends countless hours each week at the Veterans Center helping and counseling other veterans, old and young alike. He shares his experience, strength, and hope when a veteran wants to listen.

He continues to address his PTSD and alcohol dependency recovery and treatment at the VA, but now he sees his treatment in a different light. He is beginning to understand that living life is a matter of balance and that his spiritual condition is as big a part of that as is his physical and mental development. He is not running away from anything today. He is running toward new things.

Jake has joined a newly formed Vietnam Vets group at his local Veterans Center. He chooses to attend 12-step self-help meetings for his alcohol dependency. Also, he has been spending time reconnecting with Corporal Rodriquez and meeting his family for the first time.

And he has returned to that small church across the street from his apartment. He is now an usher and greeter on Sunday mornings. When the bells toll at 9:00, a whole new meaning comes with that sound. In fact, this once suicidal veteran with the wounded soul has now asked the church pastor to allow him to oversee ringing the bells on Sunday morning.

# CHAPTER 3

# Surrendering to Win

The first time I laid eyes on veteran navy pilot, LT Joe Ferguson, he was in the waiting room of our outpatient clinic in San Juan Capistrano, California. Our clinic is located not far from Naval Base San Diego and the Marine Corps' base, Camp Pendleton.

I walked over to the registration counter at one end of the waiting room to check in with the receptionist about my scheduled appointment. I picked up LT Ferguson's file. The light-yellow file folder contained a coversheet with initial information about the veteran, the referral form information, a blank Psychosocial Evaluation Worksheet, and a Determination of Level of Care form.

This appointment and time spent face-to-face with Joe Ferguson, in this first interview, would possibly be the most important turning point in Joe's life. For Joe, that time spent and the information gathered by me, his new primary therapist and addiction specialist, might mean the difference between life and death. During the next 60 minutes, the rubber would meet the road—where H2HR truly begins.

I recall thumbing through Mr. Ferguson's file, then looking up to see him seated in the corner, staring at the floor, his head propped up in his hands, his face rugged and worn. His expression was hollow and void of life. He appeared unsteady, wearing loosely fitting clothing belonging to someone else, I remember thinking.

I took a moment to study him before I made my approach and initiated the introductions. His hair was brownish blond, thinning, with receding hair lines, and cut Marine style, short on the sides, longer on top, accompanied by a week-old shadow of thick, graying facial hairs: a handsome but aging. Large bony shoulders that once supported muscle pushing through the worn fabric of his clothing. I could see the damage caused after years of abusing himself.

Although I did not know his whole story, I could nonetheless tell he had had a war going on inside; physically, emotionally, and psychologically. To an experienced eye, the trauma showed in his posture, face, and extreme lack of eye contact. I didn't have to read a file sheet of demographics and history. I felt Joe's pain from across the room. My heart was engaged. I wanted to know more.

My eyes returned to Joe's confidential file cover sheet. He had been referred to me by a social services worker at a homeless shelter in Hermosa Beach, California, a small city in Los Angeles County.

Our usual outpatient clinic intake protocol is to introduce ourselves and escort our clients to a counseling office down the hall from the waiting area. For me, this is where Heart-to-Heart Resuscitation begins: the initial greeting and the walk to my office.

I closed Joe's, file placing it under my left arm, and walked over to him. I recall, as I approached Joe, he did not move, just rolled his eyes at me, and then immediately looked back down to the floor. I could tell by the void in his eyes he was in a serious state and probably had been for quite a while.

"Mr. Ferguson, my name is Vic Montgomery, I have been asked to talk with you today to determine how we may be able to assist you. I understand a social worker by the name of Valerie called us, greatly concerned about your welfare, asking if we could see you today. Is that right, sir?"

I was now standing only a couple of feet from his chair, diagonally to his side so as not to stand over him. I waited for a response. I held out my hand to greet him, still no response. It was late in the afternoon; there was no one else in the waiting room.

A minute or so went by. I observed LT Ferguson: obvious weight loss, awkward body posture, unblinking eyes. unchanging expression. I was sensing a severely, emotionally unstable man, unable or unwilling to talk, and an inability to sit-up and look me in the eyes that indicated several possibilities of a mental disability.

"Joe, if you don't mind, I am going to sit down next to you so we can talk quietly before we go to my office. Would that be alright?"

Joe groaned quietly, "Yeah," without moving his head still cradled in his hands. I sat down in the chair next to him, giving him space.

"Joe, I know you do not know me, nor do you know what lies ahead of you. But I would like to share something with you if you are willing to listen." I paused. No response. I waited. Then, I continued without his permission.

I calmly said, "LT Ferguson, welcome home, sir. Thank you for serving our great county. I salute you, Lieutenant! And I care about what happens to you, Joe. I care if you live or die. I care that you may not know how to turn your life around right now. I care that you may feel helpless and hopeless, feelings that in the past never entered your mind. This is foreign territory for you, Lieutenant. I understand that, and I am here to help you through this, buddy, I have your six! You are a good man, LT Joe Ferguson, a TOPGUN who has lost his way, and I am going to help you find your way back if you will let me."

I risked calling him by his first name and using the personal familiar "buddy." Sometimes that backfires, but I needed to push the envelope in Joe's case— right here, right now, not tomorrow.

Joe slowly turned his face toward me, his head still in his hands and tears were streaming down his face and onto the carpet. He was about to erupt, I thought. I suspected years of pent-up emotion, maybe decades were coming to the surface.

Joe appeared to be fighting back, trying desperately not to weaken. He was twisting and turning in his seat, holding onto the arms of the chair, his bony hands grasping, turning white with strain. Joe was a man's man, trying frantically not to show any signs of weakness. Mucus and a slight tinge of blood began to dribble hanging out of his nose. His red eye veins began bulging; he was losing control. Concerned for his safety, I quickly braced his right arm and locked my left under his for support, helping him stand up. His legs were weak, and he stumbled. I grabbed him around the waist, hooking my fingers onto his belt loops and leading him slowly toward the hallway to my counseling room. At times like this, I was grateful I'm a strong six foot four and weigh 250 pounds. As we moved forward together, I motioned to the receptionist, raising my free right arm into the air, and called out the clinic code word for emergency, *Apex*.

As we proceeded down the hallway, Joe began to find his balance but could not hold back the emotions. My office door was open. Joe fell into one of my stuffed chairs, sobbing uncontrollably. I closed the door. We were alone. Joe was safe, maybe for the first time in many years. I pulled another chair next to him, sat down, and waited in silence, just being present to him. I began to listen.

It had taken all the strength Joe had left in his aging, anemic body to swing his boney legs toward the floor in a feeble attempt to roll off his urine-smelling, musky, sleeping bag lying open on the bed mattress. As he attempted to stabilize his awkward body, Joe sat upright for a moment, pausing, and then swung his feet to the floor. He immediately began rubbing his sunken eye sockets with the heels of his once powerful hands as crumbled, dry, tear-duct residue fell to the floor. His hands were shaking uncontrollably. Joe mumbled to himself, "Why did I have to wake up?"

Surveying his dimly lit, one-room apartment, Joe glanced in the direction of his peeling, 60s-something refrigerator across the room and then at a picture on the dresser next to his bed. His eyes began to moisten. Some would say they were tears. Joe could not relate. He felt dead inside. He knew he must be in hell. With blurred vision, he tried to focus on the picture. It possessed an angelic aura—it was a family picture of his wife and kids sunbathing on a sandy beach in San Diego, California. The picture was old, but time meant nothing anymore.

The small frame was tilting, falling apart, held together with a piece of faded and peeling tape. Joe grabbed the drawer, on with his skeletal right hand barely supporting him, as he rose from the bed. It took every effort to stay upright. He glanced again at the picture before him then, suddenly, crooked his head over his left shoulder in the direction of the refrigerator. He knew he had to make it to the refrigerator in order to have any chance of survival. Joe pivoted clumsily and shuffled across the small room. He was naked and stayed naked most everyday, only dressing on the rare occasions when he left his apartment. No visitors, no family came calling. —just Joe stuffed into this tiny 12'x14' mildew-smelling space, alone with his psychosis.

The 48-year-old Joe Ferguson is a decorated combat veteran, a navy pilot trained in the United States Navy Fighter Weapons School previously located at the Naval Air Station Miramar in California; more popularly known as TOPGUN. In January 1991, naval power was fundamental to the success of the Desert Storm air offensive. Lieutenant Joe Ferguson piloted an A-6 Intruder using 500-pound laser-guided bombs in "tank-plinking" strikes that mauled the enemy's armored forces.

Joe did own weapons. He kept a loaded .38 special revolver under his mattress with his old navy K-BAR utility knife. These knives used for hand-to-hand combat were carried mainly by Marine 'devil dogs' for fighting.

Joe opened the refrigerator door, his hands shaking on the handle, perspiration running down his brow onto his cheeks. Then, in desperation, he thrust his hand forward for the freezer door handle and opened it. Reaching his hand into the over-frosted freezer and grinning, he found what he had come the distance for. With no hesitation, he pulled out a pintsized glass bottle of 80-proof vodka, opened the top with his teeth, put the bottle to his chapped lips, and downed half a pint without coming up for air. Then, he wiped his mouth with his left forearm and moved to the adjacent corner of the room and slowly slid down the wall to the floorboards clutching his bottle and knees against his chest, waiting for the demons to arrive for another round of hell.

Many people do not realize there is a poisonous ingredient in alcohol called Ethanol. Ethanol poisoning is caused by drinking too much alcohol, which can lead to death.

Joe knows that! In fact, Joe is trying to kill himself. He doesn't want to wake up another morning. Joe has lost his will to face life. He has lost everything meaningful to him—family, dignity, respect and self-worth. Joe has lost sight of freedom and control, love and connection, and integrity and truth. He sees no light at the end of the tunnel. Joe Ferguson has no feeling of wellbeing. Faith, belief, and hope have all but disappeared for him. At mid-life, he was suffering a slow, lonely, and painful death from alcohol poisoning, complicated by unknown physical health problems and a severe and disabling psychiatric disorder.

Vets often feel as if they are looked down on by fellow veterans if they go into the VA for mental health services, many experiencing the feeling of being "less than"— a loss of honor. They also worry that if they have a mental illness or addiction issues, in some way that will have a negative impact on their benefits or level of service. They talk with me about the stigma of "weakness" if they go in for help.

Active duty troops have the same problems in theater. Many combat troops suffering from depression or anxiety, maybe even undiagnosed PTSD or TBI, feel that if they go in for sick call, especially during rapid combat deployment, for mental health reasons, they will be labeled as "sissy" or "crybaby" by their fire team leaders and all the way up the chain of command to their company commanders. Many career soldiers worry this may affect their rank and promotion possibilities. This stigma of not being able to complete their mission is unacceptable to many combat-hardened warriors and their leaders, even to combat mission pilots. So, they go untreated, many overly medicated, and slip through the cracks of the debriefing system, addicted, under-diagnosed, and not properly screened before, during, or after deployment.

The therapeutic value of my term, *heart-to-heart resuscitation*, is sometimes difficult to understand. Just being present with Joe that day, not needing to fill the sometimes uneasy silence with shallow words is at this moment the journey begins....connecting with Lieutenant Joe Ferguson, heart to heart.

We were together for maybe 15 minutes when my phone intercom flashed, indicating a need to call or go to the reception office. I sensed what the message likely was. The emergency alerts code, Apex, I called out to the receptionist meant for her to call 911. The police and paramedics had probably arrived. So as not to alarm Joe, I addressed him in a whisper, "Joe, we have called the paramedics just in case you need medical attention ...just as a precaution. I want to make sure you are safe. May we have them come back here to my office and check your vital signs and anything else you might need of them? Would you do that Joe? I've got your back, Lieutenant."

I clearly remember Joe looked up, then peered deeply into my eyes for the first time, and responded in a shaky voice, "What did you say your name was?"

"Vic, Joe. Vic Montgomery. I am your counselor from here on out if you want me to be."

Joe looked down at his hands, moist from the flow of tears earlier. He looked back up again, directly into my eyes, inches from my face, and, wiping the remaining moisture and mucus from his face with his forearm sleeve, replied, "Yeah, Vic, let's do this thing."

I was relieved because not all clients accept help when first asked. In Joe's case, though, I could discern he was at the end of his rope: just sick and tired of being sick and tired.

The paramedic examined Joe and then called me aside out of my office. He suggested Joe be transported to the nearest hospital emergency department for a 72-hour psychiatric hold. He also suggested a thorough medical examination.

I agreed, even without knowing all the medical or psychological facts. I thought it would be a wise thing to do: get Joe checked out and stabilized. But the real question was still looming. Would Joe Ferguson agree to go voluntarily to a hospital in an ambulance? Legally, Joe would not have to go voluntarily. However, if the police or I insisted, Joe would have to go involuntarily.

Section 5150 is the section of the California Welfare and Institutions Code that allows a qualified officer or clinician to involuntarily confine a person deemed to have a mental disorder that makes him (or her) a danger to himself and/or others and/or is gravely disabled. I recall clearly, considering that I do not want to tell Joe I have that option. I want to see how the events play out before having to make a difficult but necessary decision.

I returned to my office, closed the door for privacy and sat down next to Joe. I began in an encouraging and what I hoped was a motivating manner, "Joe, the medics suggest you go with them for a medical evaluation at a hospital not far from here. You would be there for a psychiatric observation for 72 hours and maybe more days if they recommend a medical detoxification from the alcohol in your body." I paused, facing him. There was no response—zip, zero. Joe reeked of alcohol.

I remember saying to him, "Now, Joe, before you answer me, I respectfully want to you to consider a few things. First, you already know you are ill and may be in need of medical attention. You are an intelligent man. I know you know this. You haven't been eating much at all. Joe, you have been drinking poison uncontrollably for how many years now? I smell the odor of alcohol streaming from your body. Your eyes tell me a desperate and lonely story." I paused to give Joe a moment to consider. I remember as if it were yesterday, you could cut the tension in the room with a knife. I waited for his all-important answer.

Joe glanced up at me with questioning eyes. Tears started welling up again. He sniffled heavily, attempting to contain his emotion. Joe looked away, fidgeting with his hands and symmetrically rubbing the malnourished thigh muscles of his upper legs as if to relieve some sort of pain. I saw Joe looking around my office, at the pictures I have on my wall. The direction of his head stopped abruptly as his eyes focused on a colorful red, white, and blue VA poster I had placed strategically on the wall behind my desk just for moments like this. It reads: It Takes the Courage and Strength of a Warrior to Ask for Help.

I firmly believe in always being straightforward and truthful with the vets in my program. Heart-to-Heart Resuscitation has no room for deception. Building a trusting relationship from the very beginning was paramount. In Joe's case, this may have been the very first time anyone had ever told him the truth about his addiction. I recall thinking how serious the situation had become. This crisis intervention had to be immediate.

During alcohol and other drug treatment counseling, a client's subliminal denial and dishonesty are unique roadblocks that must be addressed and replaced with acceptance and openness as quickly as possible if there is to be any opportunity for successful lifestyle changes on the long road to recovery. It doesn't matter if the individual is an honest and standup guy in his earlier life, once mind altering chemicals take over the mind, body and spirit of a person, after time, the person is left for dead. The boss at work no longer stands with them, so they lose their job; the family leaves for higher ground, and friends stop calling. The loose clothing draped over a degenerating body starts smelling, and what money is left mysteriously disappears. So it goes in the world of chemical dependency addiction. I liken it to a man standing in front of a bathroom mirror as steam begins rolling in from the shower—a steamy fog bank slowly covers the image of the man in the mirror. Then, in a matter of a heartbeat, there are no more images to see at all—the man is lost in the fog.

Joe looked at me, saying nothing. I continued to talk.

"If you agree to go into the hospital, Joe, you will be taken by ambulance from here, no sirens or lights, and checked into the emergency department where a psychiatric nurse will greet you. In fact, Joe, I will call ahead and have them waiting to admit you with a referral directly from me."

"Are you listening to me, Lieutenant?" Joe's eyes had begun to wander, and I wanted him to reconnect with me. He slowly nodded. I paused, giving Joe time to digest all this information.

After a few minutes, I continued. Joe could not or would not engage with me in this discussion. The decision I had asked him to make was a commitment. Alcoholics and drug addicts do not like to commit to anything.

"I sincerely hope you agree with this recommendation, Lieutenant, because it is a matter of life and death for you. When you complete your psychological observation and alcohol detoxification, I will be waiting for you. Joe, I have your back, buddy. I will not leave you. I will arrange for you to be picked up in our clinic van and brought back here, directly to this clinic to meet with me. I give you my word on that. Then, after we complete your initial paperwork and get your MediCal insurance and financial assistance updated, I will have housing for you at our recovery home. In fact, Joe, we will have a bed available for you when you return. How does that sound as an initial plan? Will you make a commitment to do this today?" Joe's eyes were dancing around as if he were looking for a way out of my office. I sensed his uneasiness.

Then, suddenly, there came a break in the silence, "What happens at the hospital?" Joe impulsively asked under his breath.

I responded, "Joe, the body's reaction to the removal of a substance it has become dependent on is called withdrawal. Withdrawal causes craving for more of the substance being removed, in your case alcohol. The period when your body is trying to overcome its addiction is called detoxification or detox, Joe. This is the first step in overcoming your alcohol addiction. Let me encourage you: thousands and thousands of successfully recovered chemically dependent individuals have gone before you. Detox is a huge and significant step for you to be successfully rehabilitated."

I paused, then continued, "I will be straightforward and honest with you all the time, Lieutenant. There will be withdrawal symptoms or what we call side effects when you abruptly stop drinking, especially after prolonged use. That is why we recommend a hospital stay to help you with this. Some side effects may include sweating and shaking, maybe headaches, certainly alcohol cravings with nausea, and may be even vomiting and stomach cramps. But Joe, because you are going straight to the hospital you will be under medical care, and the doctors will medically treat you with non-addictive drugs called Klonepin or Buprenophex so you will feel relief from these side effects. And Joe, generally, the time period for detox is only 3-7 days under monitored supervision. I will look in on you to see how you progress. Does that make any sense to you, Joe?"

Joe slowly nodded his head and stared forward as if in a daze. He was beginning to withdraw. We had to get him admitted immediately.

One of the most difficult things in the world for a chronic alcoholic to do is to allow someone to come between him and his bottle. So, Joe was sitting there in my counseling office, two feet away from me, having to make a very difficult decision: whether to stop drinking.

Joe shifted, squirming in the overstuffed chair he had fallen into 45 minutes before. He had not answered the question about admitting himself into the hospital. So, the silence continued. I remember thinking in a theoretical sort of way… do I reach out and come to Joe's rescue and continue to console him? No, I cannot do that. He must step up to the plate and take ownership of his condition right here, right now. I remained quiet and observed as Joe searched for the answer. The left side of his face began to twitch. His eyes darted around the room. Sweat ran down his cheeks.

Watching this combat hero struggle, I was so tempted to speak. I continued to look into his face. Do I continue to help him figure this out? No, absolutely not! *Joe Ferguson you must make this decision,* I mused.

Sometimes, as chemical dependency counselors and addiction therapists, we find ourselves wanting recovery for our clients more than they do themselves. This is not the right way to approach recovery. Alcoholics and addicts must come to a point in their first stages of rehabilitation when they say, "I'm sick and tired of being sick and tired. I want to change my life." They must take ownership of their own abstinence and compulsive out-of-control behavior for long-term recovery to work. We can't do it for them. The sooner they realize the ball is in their court the sooner their lives will begin to change.

Suddenly, like a puppet pulled up by a set of strings dangling from his shoulders, and a bit unbalanced, Joe caught himself, popped out of the chair, and said, "Vic, let's do this thing!"

I stood up about the same time and pivoted, stepping sideways to pick up the telephone receiver on the credenza behind my desk. I told the receptionist to tell the paramedics my client will be taking that ride to the emergency room.

And so it was, Joe Ferguson made the toughest decision for any alcoholic—to walk away from the bottle. Oh, this was just the beginning of a tough and long road ahead for Joe, but nevertheless this was a life changing first step. A week went by, and I visited Joe in the detox unit. I told him he has a bed waiting for him and he can look forward to beginning his new life. Joe managed a small but labored grin, obviously not the happiest camper on the medical unit.

The second time Lt. Joe Ferguson entered our clinic waiting room, I was standing there waiting to greet him with a hardy handshake and said, "Congratulations, Joe! Welcome to your new recovery program." We exchanged smiles and small talk for a couple of minutes.

Then, I moved things along and said, "Joe, if you will come back to my office. we can talk some more. I am eager to hear how it went over there at the hospital and get some paperwork completed, okay?"

Joe immediately agreed.

As we were walking down the hallway, I pointed out the location of the bathrooms and other counseling offices and then turned into group room #2. In the room was a circle of 15 light green, padded, stacking chairs, all positioned against the wooden wall guard rails along the walls. I explained to Joe that he would be attending his first group meeting that evening in that room at 6 p.m. He nodded, looking around the large square space. I saw him glance at the motivational posters hanging on the walls. He walked over to one of them. The poster is titled: Attitude. The inscription says: "The great discovery of any generation is that a human being can alter his life by altering his attitude" by William James. He turned, looked me straight in the eye, and walked to another poster that read:  Make It Happen. The inscription reads: "Greatness is not in where we stand but in what direction we are moving. We must sail sometimes with the wind and sometimes against it — but sail we must and not drift, nor lie at anchor." - Oliver Wendell Holmes.

Once again Joe paused to turn and look at me. This time, his face had a small hint of a grin on it.

I elaborated, "Joe, this group you are going to attend tonight is an orientation group designed to let all our new clients ask questions collectively and interactively and be introduced to each other. There will be discussion about the recovery program schedules, other groups, and agendas for the weeks and months ahead. I will be leading this group. Right now, there are 11 males and one female member in the group, including yourself—all combat veterans." Joe's face remained unchanged.

Joe and I turned and walked out of group room #2 and down the hallway to my office. I walked beside Joe, not in front of him or behind him, side by side, showing support and unity. This is another instance where "heart-to-heart resuscitation" shows a caring attitude and teamwork—the buddy system. It was the simple things where Joe and I began building a trusting relationship as he embarked on probably the most difficult challenge of his life: a lifetime of abstinence and a clean and sober living lifestyle.

As we sat together in my office going over Joe's psychosocial evaluation for the better part of an hour and a half, I learned many more details about the pain and destruction in Joe's life causing him to want to drink himself to death.

The evaluation began with Joe Ferguson's personal information and demographics, age, date of birth, ethnicity, veteran status and referral sources. The next section is one of the most important initial parts of the form. The question: What is the presenting problem? And what is the client's perspective on the need for treatment?" For the most part, in Joe's situation, these sections of the evaluation had already been answered. Joe's actions spoke louder than words when he agreed to put himself in medical detox.

The second and third sections of the evaluation were his medical and mental health history. When Joe returned from the hospital, he brought with him the medical records from his attending physicians. The reports indicated medical testing and blood work had been done and showed several areas of concern. Healthwise the doctor was requesting a follow up appointment as soon as possible. Joe had been diagnosed with some internal organ damage, anemia, alcohol abuse, and dependence. The mental health diagnosis from the psychiatrist was indicating Paranoid Schizophrenia and Post Traumatic Stress Disorder.

LT Joe Ferguson, naval pilot, TOPGUN, combat veteran had made a gallant attempt to survive on his own, self-medicating, without help, living on the streets at times, with co-occurring illnesses he was not aware of, nor did he take the time to find out about during his alcohol stupor. Joe was self-medicating to numb the horrific emotional and physical pain within. He learned to survive living in his private hell for a long, long time.

The next section of the psychosocial evaluation asks about family and family relationships, history, and social functioning. This is a key factor in the discovery phase of the assessment interview—a time when I get to uncover and discover more about my client's family relationship dynamic. It is a very effective tool, generally called a genogram, a graphic pictorial indicating personal family relationships and medical history.

I began by asking Joe, "Tell me about your family, Joe. Where are they living now, and what is your relationship with them today?"

Joe reached down from the chair with his right hand, wrist still tagged with the green hospital patient identification band, to a small plastic grocery bag lying on the floor tilted against his right ankle. It always remained close to him—protected. His only cherished possession left in the world. He pulled out a small, worn, framed picture of his wife and two daughters on a beach. Handing me the picture, he said, "They are all I have in the world." Joe's voice cracked, he sniffled, and his cheeks became moist, "but they are gone now. I haven't seen them in years. It was my fault they left. I drank too much and got drunk a lot, so couldn't hold down a job. My life started changing about two years after I returned home from combat in the Persian Gulf. I don't know, Vic, I just couldn't hold things together. I was having nightmares, bad dreams... haunting stuff, some about the war, seeing all those burning bodies and civilian people on fire running from bombed automobiles on the 'Highway of Death.' Vic, I slaughtered civilians with the bombs I was carrying. Flying in low, I saw blackened skeletons grotesquely twisted among charred frames of cars and trucks, their clothes, skin, and hair burnt off. It haunts me. I started to drink a lot. I drank until I got so drunk, I would pass out. That was the only way I could sleep all night. No one understands what I go through—and the guilt! A few years back, I started hearing voices no one else heard. It was awful. I didn't want to wake up in the mornings."

I listened. Joe made occasional eye contact.

"My family couldn't take my drunken, angry outbreaks anymore, so I packed up and moved to San Diego. I haven't seen my wife and kids since then." He paused and cleared his throat, "So many years now, I lost track. It was shortly after that I lost the house and went homeless, bouncing from living in my car to small, cheap inexpensive boarding houses. I finally lost my car to the police impound lot because I got my 4th DWI and lost my license...did jail time."

This weary warrior leaned forward and continued speaking in a tired tone, "I learned how to live on the streets moving from shelter to shelter, mission district to mission district, for the soup kitchens. I knew where the food banks were and the days and times churches gave out free dinners. I would hang around the outside of restaurants to get leftover food, handouts from the cooks behind the kitchens. They began to know me by my street name, Gunner. They fed me, and I told my blood-and guts-war stories."

Joe hesitated. I handed him some tissues from my side drawer. He blew his nose and wiped his eyes. He crumpled the used tissue in his hand, looking around the room for something to put it in. I got up and reached for the trash can holding it in front of him. He tossed it in. The room was silent for another short moment. I sat down.

There are moments like these in my career when my clients regurgitate their deepest, darkest secrets—their experiences learning to survive in a living hell—I will never forget…ever! How can you ever forget and profess to have a heart?

I said in a low tone, "Joe you will be joining a group of men and women tonight at 6 o'clock, in group room 2, and many of these vets saw combat on the ground in Iraq and more recently in Afghanistan. We also have a couple of Vietnam combat veterans in your group. Believe me, Lieutenant, most will understand what you went through and what you are feeling today."

"Any pilots in the group?" Joe asked with some measure of enthusiasm.

"I will let them tell their stories as I would hope you will share yours as well, Joe."

I continued, "Now we have to complete your evaluation, so please tell me about your alcohol use and other drug use and about any other treatment you have received or completed in the past."

It was necessary to dig deeper into his past to search for more information about his first use of alcohol, how regularly he drank, how much he consumed, and how long to his last drink. This information would help me confirm the diagnosis established at the hospital and help me determine what level of care I would offer Joe and my treatment plan recommendations. I was formulating a treatment plan of action as he spoke—goals to be developed over the weeks and months ahead.

Joe picked up on the cue, "I think I was rushed to the hospital ER on a couple of occasions over the years, but I honestly don't remember where or when that happened. I think I blacked out or something once and was found in an alley somewhere. Cops called an ambulance, and I ended up in a ward. Not much more to report right now on that. My memory comes and goes, you know."

I affirmed what he had shared and said, "I can understand, Joe, how you're struggling right now, but as time goes on, your memory will begin to come back to you more and more. And as your sobriety continues, and you work on your treatment plan objectives and goals, your lifestyle will also improve dramatically. And Joe, after a time, I will help you find your family."

Joe just stared at me. His eyes began to get misty. He remained in control. I continued to listen and took notes.

"I started drinking when I played football at the Naval Academy. After the games, we would party, but I hit the books pretty much during the week, not much drinking. After graduation, I enlisted into the TOPGUN navy pilot program at Miramar, California. Not much drinking there, either. We were in the air most of the time.

"Then came the Persian Gulf War in 91," Joe bellowed.

I hadn't heard him raise his voice to that level until now. Anger engulfed on his face. His cheeks reddened, and his jaws clenched.

I could instantly see the story telling had begun to overwhelm him. I didn't want to open up this infected emotional wound, at least not at this time, so I chose to move on until he was in a more stable place to talk about such traumatic experiences.

"Joe…Joe, hold on, buddy…let's visit this topic at another time. We can wrap this up, enough for today, how does that sound? Let's get you settled into your new sober living home."

Joe took a moment to regroup and responded, "Yeah, I'm tired."

That afternoon, I arranged for Joe to check into our sober living home, just walking distance from the clinic. He would be living with 22 other people, all in recovery from mind-altering chemicals, many suffering from co-occurring disorders.

Joe was provided with a large plastic laundry basket loaded with bed linens, pillow, bath towel, and a bag of personal hygiene items and was escorted to his room on the second floor. He was greeted at the door by his new roommate, Jared Murdock. Joe later was taken to a thrift store in the neighborhood to buy additional clothing. His MediCal benefits paperwork had been completed, approved, and submitted for benefits to pay for residential housing, food stamps and outpatient clinic counseling services. Our staff also assisted Joe in applying for VA benefits and SSI.

Lieutenant Ferguson settled into his new housing unit and found his bed. He was exhausted. He laid down and fell asleep.

# CHAPTER 4

# Haunting Feelings of
# Fear and Guilt

It is my experience as a primary therapist that veterans from all past and present wars and conflicts are coming forward in increased numbers with symptoms they have been living with for years, even decades. Delayed po-traumatic stress disorder problems often occur unexpectedly. Flashbacks or a sense of reliving the experiences and feelings of extreme distress when reminded of the trauma and physiological stress responses to reminders of the incidents (throbbing heart, quickness in breathing, stomach queasiness, muscle tension or sweating) are disturbing memories of and reactions to the traumatic event resulting in bad dreams about the insidious encounter. These distressing symptoms can emerge at anytime, anywhere—sometimes out of the blue. At other times, they are triggered by something that reminds the veteran of the original traumatic event: a noise, an image, certain words, or even a smell. Through Hanna's story, I pointed-out suggested methods for overcoming these haunting feelings of fear and guilt.

Hanna was an Air Force combat pilot, living with a 100% service-connected disability: post-traumatic stress disorder. Increasing her disability, she felt guilty for contributing to the deaths of so many innocent Iraqi civilians. She called the clinic sobbing heavily; her noisy, forced breathing made it difficult to understand her on the telephone.

Her whimpering voice began, "I am shaking and wrapped around my best friend in the world." She sniffled, "My dog." The combat veteran went on to say fireworks were too much for her. She was on prescribed medication from the VA every day, but storms, sonic booms from the F-14 jets at the nearby Air Force Base, and most anything noisy and sudden startled her. The Independence Day fireworks' loud bangs and whistles over and near her house triggered too much of her past experiences as a bomber pilot. "Too many memories and flashbacks," she said and began to cry. PTSD has become a significant disability that was identified during the Vietnam War as Adjustment Disorders and later renamed PTSD.

Today, PTSD affects approximately 30% of the veterans who served in Desert Shield/Storm and the Iraq and Afghanistan Wars. Research has found that trauma from military combat produces a profound sense of alienation and alarm and causes questioning of basic life assumptions that one's environment is physically and psychologically safe. Hanna did not feel safe. In fact, she kept the lights on in her house when she slept.

"I am dreadfully afraid of thunder and lightning when the summer storms come. I cannot fly in airplanes anymore. My life is over. Give me two reasons why I should live. I find myself avoiding all social activity, and most of the time recently I feel numb and nervous. I think I am depressed. I cry often, sometimes daily. If it weren't for my 15-year-old dog, I wouldn't be on the phone today talking to you. I know how to kill myself. I am an American combat pilot," Hanna relayed.

As I spoke with Hanna and reassured her that I was there to support her, not judge her, she began to open up and dry her tears. Lieutenant Hanna Bonnar shared she was a combat bomber pilot at the beginning of Operation Desert Storm, an offensive campaign that was originally designed to enforce the United Nation's resolutions that Iraq must cease its rape and pillage of its weaker neighbor Kuwait and withdraw its forces from the small country. She remembered a message delivered to the command on January 16, 1991 by General H. Norman Schwarzkopf, Commander in Chief of U.S. Central Command. Hanna said she memorized his short message: "My confidence in you is total. Our cause is just! Now you must be the thunder and lightning of Desert Storm. May God be with you, your loved ones at home, and our country."

Hanna continued to reveal to me her experiences in the war. She recalled that the day after the general's opening message on January 17, Desert Storm began with a coordinated attack that included Tomahawk land attack missiles launched from cruisers, destroyers, and battleships in the Persian Gulf and Red Sea. The missile launches opened a carefully crafted joint strategic air campaign. The initial barrage of over 100 missiles took out heavily defended targets in the vicinity of Baghdad and made a critical contribution to eliminating Iraqi air defenses and command and control capabilities.

During those early hours of the war, Hanna recalled, "I contributed to the destruction of Iraq's air and naval forces, anti-air defenses, ballistic missile launchers, communications networks, electrical power, and more. I joined the joint and allied partners in inflicting violent military losses with precision bombing from our high-tech aerial weaponry. As full partners in that campaign, we as Navy and Marine Corps aviators flew from carriers and amphibious ships in the Red Sea and Persian Gulf and from bases ashore from the day hostilities began until the cease-fire was ordered." Hanna paused.

I know about PTSD. Avoidance through emotional numbing anxiety and depression is most common. The signs were all there. I waited.

Then, she began speaking again. "Umm ...from 'H-hour' when the air campaign began," she whispered, "until the end of offensive combat operations 43 days later, I helped obliterate key targets and helped ensure the United States military and its coalition partners owned the skies over Iraq and Kuwait. I have had to learn to live with this painful memory and the thought I could be responsible for the deaths of innocent people, women, and children. My thoughts are intense at times. I feel irritable, and I can't concentrate. I experience life-like daydreams of certain scary experiences that return repeatedly and haunt me—and, Oh, my! the nightmares! I can't take this anymore," she said with a keen sense of sadness.

I listened intently. I marveled how specific she was with every detail; at the same time, I felt a broken heart. A wave of helplessness washed over me. My stomach tightened, and my heart began to pound. I am a professional interventionist. I know how to treat such emotional wounds. It just hurts the very essence of my being to witness such a good person go through such agony, This is a good woman, a fine veteran pilot desperate to be forgiven for deeds for which she felt guilty. I felt Hanna was going through the feelings of seeing her life as an unconnected, distinct separation of emotions. I heard it in her words. Clinically, I would say these symptoms are the separation of a group of usually connected mental processes, such as emotion and understanding, from the rest of her mind. In translation, she was reliving the trauma of combat through dissociation. At that moment, she felt the only way to separate her from all that misery was by ending her life.

Dissociation is a normal response to trauma and allows the mind to distance itself from experiences that are too much for the psyche to process at that time. Dissociative disruptions can affect any aspect of a person's functioning.

"Hanna, will you let me help you?" I asked after she stopped speaking. There was nothing but silence. "Hanna, I will not leave you. We are in this together. I care about what happens to you. I can get you the help you need. I will see to it. You took the first big step in helping yourself today, Hanna, you found this number and called it! Oh, yes, you do have a reason to live, and I will give you more than two reasons why if you will let me!" I paused, then began again, calmly, "I know you are still on the line. Please talk to me. Lieutenant. Have you done anything to hurt yourself today?: I pleaded for a response. I know Hanna is crying out for help because she made the call; but if she made the call after taking some pills or cutting herself, this could be tragic.

"I am so hurt," she quietly began talking again. "I am not a killer. I had no idea I would feel this way. I am guilty of slaughtering innocent women and children. I can't sleep in my own house. I can't work. I already see doctors. I am on medications every day. What else is there? I feel hopeless. What is there to live for?"

"Hanna, have you hurt yourself? Please, talk to me," I insisted. "I want to get you some help, but I need to know where you live so we can come to you right now." I was thinking I might have to call the sheriff for a welfare check; the signs were classic:

> Persons who believe they are trapped in a situation with no possible solution and no resources to bear the mounting anguish are seriously depressed. Suicidal preoccupation soon follows such a conviction. The expression of hopelessness is a sensitive indicator of suicidal intent (Victoroff, 1983).

Hanna needed help and quickly! The police and fire department had been alerted by me alerting my office staff and were en route. They had located Hanna's home by tracing her phone number from the caller ID on our phone. Now, I waited. Hanna was not responding on the phone. My responsibility was to get her to safety. My thoughts raced. These are the toughest moments of my job.

## Identifying Suicidal Signs and Symptoms

Here are some of the warning signs, "silent" signals, and personality characteristics that alert you to when a veteran close to you might consider life too tough to face.

- Feelings of not belonging; a difficult time connecting in relationships and bonding with others
- Social isolation: not participating in the social community
- Continually expressing feelings of helplessness, worthlessness, hopelessness
- Survivor's guilt: "It should have been me" or "It is my fault my buddy died"
- Feelings of being trapped
- Not taking prescribed medications for psychiatric disorders such as anxiety and depression
- Physical pain that is unbearable with little hope of relief
- Family history of suicide or depression; a fellow veteran's suicide
- Prior suicide attempts
- Untreated medical problems, such as PTSD and TBI, that go undetected or unreported
- Covered-up rage that is acted upon from time to time
- Living with a constant negative attitude: everything past, present, and future is bleak
- Possessing the lethal means to follow through with suicide
- Pre-existing conditions of major disorders, such as PTSD, TBI, depression, alcohol or drug abuse, schizophrenia, and paranoid personality disorder.

Some disorders can trigger a veteran's suicide even if medications, under treatment, are being taken. Research and media reports indicate that a significant number of veteran suicides happen while under doctor's care. Such signs and red flags can occur even when veterans, who have gone in for counseling and therapy have themselves realized the impossibility of forgetting their combat experiences and have recognized their hopelessness. I usually advise my clients that they should attempt to banish all thoughts of war from their minds after they share their stories; they should look forward, not backward. I firmly believe in heart-to-heart resuscitation: a genuine, caring and spiritually loving attitude toward every veteran, encouraging, motivating, and coaching traumatized combat veterans to visualize pleasant thoughts far, far away from the combat zones. As many veterans know, "Living with a chronic illness, physical, mental or both, adds to the normal pressure of everyday life. This can lead to feelings of anxiety or stress."

## Techniques to Manage Anxiety

It is important that veterans are taught basic techniques to help them manage their feelings and anxious situations and to avoid additional stress and negative health effects. It is also important that veterans remember that the VA doctor or healthcare provider is the single best source of information regarding veterans' health. They should be encouraged to consult their doctor or healthcare treatment team if they have any questions about their health or any of their medications.

The following are some helpful strategies I share for getting beyond troubling symptoms and relieving stress, depression, and anxiety. The most common ways to relieve stress and anxiety are breathing exercises and muscle relaxation; other techniques include visualization, total desensitization, positive thinking, storytelling, and spirituality. Here is a summary of suggested techniques:

*Breathing Exercises*

I tell veterans to begin by sitting or lying in a comfortable position. Then:

- take a deep breath, feeling their abdomen expand;
- exhale by drawing your lips together at the sides to form a circle (this allows prolonging and regulating breath);
- while exhaling, feel their abdomen deflate and shoulders relax.

They should take two or three deep breaths in this manner.

Once they become proficient, they can begin using this breathing technique when they experience stressful situations and should practice daily to relieve everyday stress.

## Muscle Relaxation

Tense, strained muscles are a common effect of stress. I suggest a way to relax muscles by

- sitting or lying in a comfortable position;
- Then, taking a deep breath and slowly tighten and relax muscle groups—hands, feet, arms, legs, chest, shoulders, and abdomen—in succession; and
- exhaling before relaxing.

Repeat as many times as comfortable.

## Visualization

This technique, sometimes called reframing (Rogers, 1959),[3] has veterans assign mental representations to their negative feelings and then change those images into positives. For example, if they experience anger about a physical limitation, they can learn to connect that angry feeling with the color red. Then, in their mind, they can slowly try to turn the red into a color they associate with a peaceful feeling, such as green. They can also try adding music and artwork to enhance the relaxation benefits of visualization.

## Total Desensitization

In counseling, combat veterans are often asked to prioritize a list of stress-producing events such as exercise, travel, mixing with family, etc. Have the veterans create their own list. Suggest that they concentrate on the least stressful activity on the list during a state of relaxation until they feel comfortable with it. Once you attain a comfortable feeling with it, they repeat the process with the next item on the list and continue in this manner through all the items.

## Positive Thinking

This technique is like visualization, but instead of images, it focuses on changing negative thoughts to positive ones. As veterans to take a moment to reflect on negative thoughts they've had recently or recurring negative thoughts they have. Once they identify these thoughts, they will also begin to identify

---

3. Rogers speaks of internal "frames of reference" that refer to an individual's unique view of the world and how it impacts him/her.

negative thoughts as they have them. They should take time to address these negative thoughts and turn them into positive ones. For example, instead of saying, "I probably can't walk too far without losing my breath and panicking," they might say, "I can relax and take a 5-minute walk."

*Storytelling*

Deena Metzger (2002) suggests that an important part in a veteran's healing process includes storytelling. Likewise Edward Tick (2005) suggests in his writing that the efficacious counselor and facilitator should always encourage "digging deep" with their clients in order to uncover the real story details and emotions and work to transfer the moral weight of the experiences from the individual to the community. Without a good facilitator, a survivor might endlessly repeat details of an event but not experience the release of related emotions, the accurate recording of history, or the making of meaning—all of which are essential in the recovery from post-traumatic stress.

*A Spiritual Journey*

People are spiritual beings. We have souls as well as flesh and bones. We all are special in the eyes of God. The Bible says we are made in the image of God. How amazing is that? Whatever a veteran's belief right now, a power greater than us all can be sought, and learning to pray is where the discovery begins. It is here where life begins again for my distressed combat veterans with wounded souls. Right here the suffering, tormented soul can find relief and a reason to live. My technique of heart-to-heart resuscitation provides a safe environment that lays these important foundations and helps veterans prepare for a renewed spirit wanting to embrace life once again. Expect a miracle.

Most counselors have experienced cases of combat mania especially in the form of neurosis emanating from anxiety. We are faced with the problem of what advice to give concerning the attitude the veteran should adopt toward his or her war experience. Generally, the primary goals of all crisis intervention therapists, nurses, counselors, and clinical social workers are not to provide veterans with over-the-telephone therapy or tele-psychiatry. A clinician's mission is to get the veterans to safety. In fact, each crisis should be handled with extreme priority that includes immediate intervention advice and heart-to-heart interviewing and assessment. The caller must then be stabilized and/or rescued by the police and emergency medical team and in many cases, with an emergency room stay for psychiatric evaluation and consultation follow-up. The most chronic cases will require immediate hospitalization and an assigned behavioral health treatment team.

So it was with Hanna. Hanna would see me for an intake assessment and consultation appointment at our outpatient clinic after the hospital discharge, but right now we were on the phone together. I was waiting for the report of her condition by the on-site first responder team that is always instructed to call back the referring medical provider. I waited. No word. No one picked up the receiver. I felt uneasy, so I placed a call.

"Hello, this is Sergeant Bill Williams," a voice barreled over the phone. I held Hanna's line open all that time I was speaking with the sergeant. I had promised her I would never leave her. I felt a heart-to-heart connection.

"Hello, Sergeant Williams, this is Vic Montgomery I made the rescue call for the veteran, Lieutenant Hanna Bonnar. How is our veteran Hanna doing?" I asked, worried about her welfare.

"What is your name again, who are you?" the sergeant asked, questioning my authority to be involved.

"Vic Montgomery. I work as a therapist for vets here in town. Hanna is one of our vets. Please handle her with care, officer, she is a combat pilot war veteran. Will you do that for me?"

"It is being done as we speak, Mr. Montgomery" the police officer replied. "The EMTs are here already and attending to her. It appears she is unconscious, sitting in a chair with the telephone in her lap. Her vital signs are irregular, but the paramedics say she will be alright—pill overdose, they think. We got here just in time."

I found out later the police had had to break a window to enter the home and had found Hanna slumped in the chair by the phone. After finding out Hanna was safe, I put my receiver down on my desk and walked briskly down the hall. As I made my way, I said a prayer of thanks for whatever help God had given me to get this vet to safety. Hanna needed to find out how to administer self-care and learn how to forgive and let go. Beginning with herself. This courageous combat pilot had to learn how to heal her feelings of having done wrong and realize the purpose for which she served was courageous and meaningful for her country—and for other countries of the world.

Hanna receives specialized care for her condition with me, at our clinic. We see each other at 6 o'clock on Tuesdays and Thursdays with the other veterans in group room # 2,

# CHAPTER 5

# A Mother and Her Son

Elsie Murdock found herself staring out the living room window for hours at a time, not moving a muscle or shifting a limb, just sitting in the living room of her small farmhouse, rocking in her old chair, staring far-far away. The same rocking chair where she had nursed and rocked to sleep in her arms her first and only child many years go. In that same rocker, she spent endless days and countless late nights sewing clothes and knitting booties, scarves and winter caps for her only son, Jared.

In his early years, Jared was a rough-and-tumble, fearless young man, large and husky for his age but well-mannered and respectful—a true Murdock. Many Murdocks who had arrived from Scotland settled along the east coast of North America in communities that would go on to become the backbone of the young nation of the United States.

Jared worked with his daddy on the farm, learning the ways of hard work and the truths about nature. When Jared turned 15-years-old, his father Gavin bought him his first rifle and taught him how to hunt. Jared was a good shot. In fact, for practice, with his .22 long rifle, at 50 yards he once knocked over 10 soda cans off an old split-rail fence in a row.

As the years slipped by, Mom and Pop Murdock began showing more and more gray in their hair and slowing down a bit. Jared noticed and started picking up extra chores around the farm. He was a good young man, and his parents were very proud of him.

On Jared's 18th birthday, he was recruited by a local Marine Corps Gunnery Sergeant right out of high school. Gavin and Elsie were somewhat worried because there were rumors around town of a war brewing in Iraq, but they were too proud and patriotic to disagree with Jared's enthusiasm and courage. So, off to Parris Island, South Carolina Marine Corps boot camp training he went on a bus with eight other new recruits. Deep down, Gavin was very proud his son enlisted with the Marines because he was a former "Leatherneck" himself.

In fact, Gavin Murdock had served with the 1st Marine Division, 7th Marines in 1965 and "booted-up" in the first major engagements for American ground troops in South Vietnam.

Then, in March of 1966, the 1st Marine Division Headquarters was established at Chu Lai. By June, the entire division was in South Vietnam. Its operations included the southern two provinces of Quang Tin and Quang Ngai. Between March 1966 and May 1967, the division conducted 44 combat operations. In these operations, 1st Marine Division units decisively defeated the enemy. During the 1968 Tet Offensive, the division was involved in fierce fighting with both Viet Cong and North Vietnamese Army elements. It successfully beat back and destroyed every enemy assault in its area of operations, pursuing the enemy into its sanctuaries. It was during this period that the division received its seventh and eighth Presidential Unit Citations. Jared and his dad rarely spoke about their combat experiences.

Well, the rumors in town buzzing around the local barbershop were right. Jared shipped out a few weeks later with the 1st Marine Division 5th Marines, one of the two major U.S. land forces that participated in the 2003 invasion of Iraq.

Jared was consistent, at first writing short, restrained letters to his parents with current news about himself and the war. During a counseling session after Jared died, Elsie read me a letter Jared had written her from the war zone. I recall she paused as if to collect her thoughts, glanced up over the edge of the ragged letter she was holding for a moment, and then began to read in a soft, nostalgic tone.

Mom and Dad,

*Hi, there! How are my parents doing? Hope ok. How is ol' Jersey cow doing? Probably missin' me, pulling her udders. Ha! Dad, you can probably get Ronnie down the road to help you with the milkin'. He can use a couple extra bucks in his pocket. Well, here I am, missin' you all back home. Mom, I sure can taste those hot biscuits and gravy and ham and eggs—all of that, Ha! My C-rations sure don't compare. A lot happening again today. Just hunkering down near an old rusty metal building we just cleared. Just trying to stay alive. A couple guys in our unit got hit and were air lifted out. That keeps it real for me. We may stay awhile, waiting for more word from HQ. The latest: our division fought through the Rumaila oil fields 2 days ago, then moved north on the Iraq Highway. My rifle company fought our way to Baghdad.*

Elsie looked up again, directly into my face, locking her misty gray-blue eyes with mine, then continued reading; her strained voice trembled.

*Our division covered 808 kilometers in 17 days of bloody combat, door to door, house to house, fire fight to fire fight. I can't even share some of the stuff I see, Mom, Pop, just can't find the words. I'm ok though, just real tired. Hard to sleep sometimes. Medic gave me some meds. Had some close misses from sniper fire yesterday, a couple of mortar round and RPGs today—a lot of that, but please, don't worry, Mom. I'm tough. Oorah! I was told today that what we are doing is the deepest penetrating ground operation in Marine Corps history. It's tough stuff. Gotta go, folks.*

*Love you both,*
*Your son!*

For actions during the war, the 1st Marine Division warriors were awarded its 9th Presidential Unit Citation. This was the first of several combat citations and ribbons Corporal Jared Murdock was awarded over two tours. Post-traumatic stress was beginning to dig at his soul.

Elsie is sitting this day, wrought with melancholy as she pictures her little boy's face, thinking about their good times together while he was growing up. Her mind strolls without destination while she stares out through the colonial window grids of her large picture window facing the once occupied horse pasture of the Gavin and Elsie Murdock Farm. Elsie sits quietly evoking memories of her late husband Gavin. Her mind drifts to a place… *when her last remaining true friend and companion had died in her arms never, never ever to return to them again…never, ever, and ever…oh, so final. He would never again hold her in his strong arms and rub her aching shoulders with his large strong hands at night before bedtime or fix things around the house, just putzing.*

Elsie stayed by her husband and soul mate until his last breath. She kissed his lips and cheeks with youthful passion knowing it would be their last—and held on to him tightly until the very end. They made a pact. They were going to die together in each other's arms—neither left behind, neither to have to face the burden and fear of having to endure aging alone.

The devoted lover and bride of so many years cried out to God, "Take me, too. Lord! I have no reason for living now. There is nothing left. You have taken the love of my life, my secret strength, my bounty, my man." Elsie couldn't tear herself away from Gavin's lifeless body for hours. Mixed emotions of outrage, abandonment and resentment permeated her very soul.

That day at the hospital, Elsie Murdock felt she had no more love to give. No more children to raise, no one to cook for, and no husband to fuss over. This once confident, jubilant woman now had to go it alone—a sensation she had never anticipated. She was all about her gentle giant of a man. He was the rock in her life, the lover in her bed, and the father of her son.

Murdock was the first to help his neighbors. He was well liked by the men at his job of 32 years. Gavin was a man's man—burley and bold—a former Marine. He was the type of guy who would jump into a flaming building to save a stranger trapped inside. Yet, he was tender, a godly man who wasn't afraid to cry.

*Jared was like his daddy*, Elsie thought.

Today and many days now, Elsie experiences feelings of numbness and desperation that engulf her. As she sits, a shiver of emptiness chills body. She pulls her knitted shawl up over her shoulders.

Gavin Murdock and Elsie Ainsworth married and had their baby boy, living a happy life to the fullest, as youthful, euphoric adventurers decades ago. Now, both her men are gone.

Today, Elsie struggles with reoccurring questions. *How do I learn to live with the fact our son is dead? How can I learn to wash away the agony of this devastating loss of my own flesh and blood? Isn't a son supposed to outlive his parents? Why has God chosen for me to endure such a thing?*

Shock and disbelief reflect in her face as she rocks in silence. Her wide-open eyes reveal small, moist, globes of sadness, then become a watery reservoir of undulating tears that begins to overflow. Her high, distinctive cheek bones, void of any powder or color this day, writhe with emotion, wet with tears. Flood gates open, and tears run freely as she sits alone, embroidered hankie in hand, powerless and heavy hearted. Elsie Murdock's head is now leaning back against the rocker's padded head rest, her eyelids becoming heavier and heavier until they slide closed, cutting off the flow of ears. Moisture gathers around the seal and entanglement of her eye lashes.

Elsie's random thoughts surface again as she sleeps, the deep orange and red spikes of the sun setting on the distant rolling hills outside the window. Elsie is now deep in resting REM sleep that she has needed for days. The devoted wife and mother cries out to God, "Take me, too, Lord. I have no reason for living now. There is nothing left. You have taken my husband and now my only child. Take me now, please! How frightened I feel! I miss my boy. I miss my husband. I can't go on with this hole in my heart."

A few hours pass, and Elsie stirs, then opens her eyes. The sun has disappeared behind the shadowed wooden rolling landscape miles away from outside Elsie's window. The night has stolen in. The family room is dark. The only noise is the creaking of her wooden rocker.

This once confident, jubilant woman now must go it alone. She lost her loving husband the year earlier to cancer, exposing her to the feelings of loss she never anticipated. And now Jared, the pride and joy in her life.

As aging parents grow older and stand at the proverbial retirement-age door, if there is such a thing today, they sometimes begin to feel as if their children do not have time for them anymore. Family visits become rare. For Elsie, her family is gone. Visits from her son coming home from the Marine Corps, taking a well-deserved leave after another tour in theater, would never happen again.

There is a period, as we grow older, that painful memories and recollections are sometimes pushed aside. Some of those memories can be the upsetting ones we do not want to revisit. But for Elsie Murdock there is one memory that punishes her and doesn't go away: the thoughts of her son Jared dying tragically.

There are many questions about Jared's life that remain a mystery. For Elsie Murdock, the toughest question of all has yet to be answered. How does a mother learn to live with the fact her son committed suicide in the home where he was born and raised? Jared Murdock, age 27, U.S Marine Corps, decorated combat veteran, hung himself from the basement rafters of their home on the Murdock family farm.

I recall when Jared first walked into our clinic a couple of years after he was honorably discharged from the Marine Corp. He indicated he had served two consecutive 13-month tours with the 1st Marine Division, 1st Battalion, and 5th Marines—Operation Iraqi Freedom. His job: Warrior. His mission: scouting the dangerous roads for insurgents and killing them.

He shared this information with me in detail during our private counseling sessions and group encounters. Navy doctors had prescribed him antidepressants while in the war zone because unrelenting battle fatigue anxiety and depression prevented him from sleeping. He told me that, with no replacement rifle squads coming, many of the men of his rifle squad had to be medicated to continue their assault missions, and, fact, their search and destroy fire team didn't sleep for consecutive days while in persistent pursuit of an elusive enemy.

Jared had become 'hooked' on antidepressants to function, every day in Iraq; the drugs helped him to cope with the anxiety and the stress of combat. Speaking of the time toward the end of his tour, he had said, "I felt helpless and hopeless. I saw no relief in sight. Vic, I'm in a black hole of emptiness. I am hurting."

Jared was referred to me by a local community hospital mental health clinician who knew I was the outpatient clinic's addiction specialist primarily counseling combat veterans in the area. The referral reports passed on to me indicated Jared was found by friends, sitting in the dark of another friend's apartment, rambling to himself, acting bewildered and disoriented, and experiencing the sensation of insects crawling under his skin.

At the time Jared first came to see me, and after lab drug screening and assessments, he self-disclosed his uncontrollable use of the methamphetamine. Apparently, when the Marine corporal discharged stateside, some buddies getting out with him introduced him to snorting meth for a more immediate relief from the gloominess and depression he was experiencing. He was buying the stimulant illegally on the streets in the cities and towns; even around his farming community he could find a connection.

Methamphetamine abusers can display several psychotic features, including paranoia, visual and auditory hallucinations, and delusions. Chronic methamphetamine abuse significantly changes how the brain functions, with self-inflicted injuries being a concern. Noninvasive human brain imaging studies have shown alterations in the activity of the dopamine system that are associated with reduced motor skills and impaired verbal learning.

Recent studies of chronic methamphetamine abusers have also revealed severe structural and functional changes in areas of the brain associated with emotion and memory which may account for many of the emotional and cognitive problems I observed torturing Jared Murdock.

I recall vividly Jared describing his feelings when first beginning to use meth as an intense euphoria, a "rush" that relieved him from the thoughts of the culture shock he first went through in country and the blood and guts of his war experiences.

He could not forget the order his fire team got after a nighttime firefight to move back out and collect the mutilated enemy dead. When Jared and his buddies arrived, they discovered that some of the blooded bodies were still alive. "It was ugly," he said. "You don't always know who the bad guys are. Which one was going to cut my throat when my back is turned while I was dragging the bodies away?"

Another discussion stands out for me. Jared described the first time he kicked in a door of a small house in Bagdad, searching for terrorists. The very first thing he saw when he entered the house in a crouched and ready to kill position, lying right in front of him on the dirt floor, was a baby doll, toys, kid's shoes, and clothing spread around. The culture shock was unbearable for this farm boy. His first thought was, *what happened to these innocent children*? Jared later told me, feelings like that started affecting him a lot more than he thought they should.

One Tuesday evening, as I was standing just outside of Group Room #2 greeting our veterans as they began to file in, engaging each participant with a greeting, or handshake, fist-bump, or shoulder slap, I realized someone was missing.

"Anyone see Jared?" I interrupted the small talk, looking in the direction of the empty chair. "Let's give it a couple of minutes he may be running late."

Jimmy suddenly sat forward in his seat, twisting in my direction, "Jared doesn't say much Vic; hard to get him to talk—not sure what he was thinking or how I could help him."

I acknowledged Jimmy, nodding my head. Many in the group had puzzled looks. Danny Barnes shifted in his chair, staring from across the room at the empty chair, where Jared Murdock should be sitting. He looked back at me. We locked eyes for a moment. I could see the wear and tear on his face around his eye lids, a few old, faded scars here and there on his tight, sun-tanned skin covering his stiff face and raised cheeks—the look of a Marine you don't mess with but want on your team in a firefight.

"Vic…," Danny started in a low sharp address in my direction. "What the hell…I thought we were supposed to be accountable here—part of our program—and coming to group on time is one of those requirements, right? Hell, a man late to a fire fight may get everyone killed exposing a flank. Come on!"

"You are right, Danny. The group will hold him accountable when he gets here. You can hold the inquisition. We will begin in another couple of minutes," I said, enforcing the precept.

No Jared.

A few minutes passed, then Jimmy piped up, "Well, group, what do we do now? We leave no man behind. Yo! Do we have his phone number, Vic?"

I looked around the room at everyone. "Yes, I do, in his file folder in my office. I am the only one with access—confidentiality regs. I will get his number, give him a shout out, and see if he is okay. I will be right back so you all start group without me with your weekly check-ins. I will jump in when I get back."

I headed to my office. I plopped down onto my desk chair, reaching over and opening the file drawer on the right. I found Jared's primary phone number and made the call.

Ring. No answer. I waited a couple of moments and tried again. Hmmm…no voice mail? I opened his file again and looked for the number he entered on his information sheet for emergency contact. The number belong to his mother, Elsie Murdock. I dialed it.

"Hello, Mrs. Murdock? This is Vic Montgomery over at the clinic. How are you today?"

"I'm doing all right, Mr. Montgomery. What can I do for you?"

"Well, we were wondering if Jared is all right; he never came to group tonight and didn't call in to miss group."

Elsie's tiny voice responded wispily, "Jared hasn't been around today, Vic; not sure where he went off to?"

"Well, not to be alarmed, Mrs. Murdock. Just checking. Thank you for taking my call. Sorry to bother you. Goodbye." I hung up.

I put things away in my desk and returned to group room #2.

No Jared Murdock. *He usually is accountable.*

I sat down. "Group, just reporting in...family does not know where he is, either. No Jared."

A couple days passed. No Jared. Finally, the sheriff came by the clinic and reported that Jared had been found dead by his mother, hanging from a ceiling rafter in the Murdock family home.

Elsie Murdock called me a day after the sheriff dropped by, knowing I had counseled Jared on several occasions after he was discharged from the Marine Corps. However, she did not know, unless Jared told her, the nature of why he was in therapy. More than likely, she had no idea about his drug abuse.

Elsie asked if it would be possible to talk with me about her son and his death. She said she was battling with unanswered questions looming in her mind and unable to move on. Feeling stuck and helpless, she confided, "I breakout crying unexpectedly, sometimes uncontrollably, staring out the window for hours at a time." I sensed in her tone she was experiencing feelings of unreality, loneliness, anger, and vulnerability—symptoms of grief. I replied that I do counsel family members of veterans and would be happy to meet with her.

The first time I met Elsie Murdock in person, I walked out into the clinic waiting room and observed a petite, attractive, gray-haired woman, hair combed tightly in a bun on the upper back of her head. She was dressed fashionably in a red-and-white plaid, western-style, summer skirt. Her hands folded in her lap, she held a braided handkerchief and was looking away when I approached her. *This has got to be Mrs. Murdock,* I thought.

I greeted her, "Mrs. Murdock, how nice to meet you. I am Vic Montgomery."

"Oh...Mr. Montgomery, hello," Her head jerked forward, her face and eyes appearing a bit startled, as she glanced in my general direction.

I held my hand out to help her up and shook her tiny hand. "Mrs. Murdock, I didn't mean to surprise you. I am sorry."

"That's all right. I was simply reading the sign on your wall over there," She nodded in the direction of the water cooler. A large, printed sign hung over the cooler water bottle: Suicide Prevention Lifeline…1-800-273-8255…if you're in an emotional crisis…press 1 for Veterans.

"Can I get you anything? A cup of water?"

"No, thank you, not right now."

I studied her eyes as she looked at me. They were sad eyes. A bit blood shot and aggravated from wiping tears away. I could understand. She had the eyes of grief.

It was not long ago her son walked these hallways. Jared was in my group of 12. I can't forget the struggle he had justifying his killing in Iraq. He had a difficult time deprogramming the scenes of war from his mind and turned to drugs to relieve the pain. His dreams and memories haunted him. The pools of blood and the war-scarred landscape in Iraq clouded his mind. Jared Murdock was fighting for his life, the battle back home.

I was attempting to help and encouraged Jared to live a drug free life. I was beginning to teach him and the other men and women in the Group of 12 how to utilize the therapeutic technique of visualization described in the previous chapter. I have found visualization to be highly successful in helping turn around the lives of many combat hardened warriors addicted to drugs.

Visualization therapy completely changes the way the combat vet thinks. The veteran will no longer see himself or herself in terms of drinking or using drugs. This kind of therapy helps to alter the mental picture from that of a killer back to family man or woman (in Jared's case, on the farm). This is not an easy task, but accomplished, it changes the vet's reality through understanding and altering the underlying pictures of self.

This therapy helps to desensitize the triggers for drug cravings in the case of war zone "blood-and-guts" images and traumatic experiences. It greatly helps in personal growth as well: recreating a veteran's "clean" self and managing underlying emotional distress, depression, and trauma.

Jared and every one of the veterans in my group of 12 struggled daily to abstain from using mind-altering chemicals. That is the addictive reality of alcohol and other drugs. Some never find the answers. Others do and move on with their lives.

I walked with Elsie back to my office. Again, as with all my clients I walked side by side, showing solidarity and harmony. I wanted to demonstrate even before we sat down in my counseling room that I was standing with her through this difficult time. Not ahead of her or behind her but *with* her, side by side.

Heart-to-heart resuscitation reveals a counselor's true colors. Is the counselor *present* with the client or not? It is the only way I have found, after 20 years in this field, to earn the complete respect, trust, and confidence it takes to allow the client to open up and begin to discover the inner workings of their very being mind, body and spirit. It was only then that I found the answers Elsie was looking for.

Elsie carefully sat down in my overstuffed, burgundy colored chair. I pulled up a chair in front of her. I looked into her eyes, but before I had a chance to speak, Elsie's pent-up emotions released a myriad of questions. "I should have known my son was in trouble. It is my fault he is not living today. I knew something was wrong and did nothing about it. Is it my fault? Jared was not himself for the last year or so. He would lock himself in his room for days at a time, not eat with me, and raise his voice in anger when I asked him questions. He never used to get upset with me. I think he was drinking or something. He would wake up in the middle of the night yelling. His bedroom was upstairs at the other end of the hall from mine, so I did not hear what he was saying, but I was afraid. So, I didn't look in on him or ask anything about it. Was that the wrong thing to do? One day, I asked him what was wrong, and he got mad. So, I didn't ask any more. Things were normally peaceful around our house. Then, his father died of cancer. It was about that time I began to see changes in my son. Gavin was not there to help me. I didn't know what to do. Am I a bad mother? What should I have done? I knew something was wrong and did nothing about it. If his father were alive, he would have investigated it. Now, I've lost my only son. I feel so terrible!"

Elsie paused breathing heavily, taking a breath, blotting her eyes with her hankie as she began to weep. My heart melted.

I remember that day so clearly. The cloud of pain filled the room. I remember thinking, *I must hold my ground as a professional and not show sympathy, I cannot give her a hug even though I wanted to unless she asked for one.* These are professional therapeutic protocols we learned in Clinical Psychology Graduate school. We must keep our boundaries.

Nevertheless, I took her hands in mine and looked into her eyes. "Mrs. Murdock, we are going to find these answers for you. You are not alone anymore. I will stand with you until you feel safe and find peace and understanding of what lead to the tragic, premature death of your son and the loss of your husband, also a vet. Will you give me the opportunity to work with you on this?"

Elsie looked over her hankie and said, "You can call me Elsie."

I responded, "Please call me Vic, Elsie."

Wiping her eyes, Elsie nodded. And so it was, H2HR began that day. That first day we talked for well over an hour. I briefly covered the stages of grief and the feelings associated with them. I validated how she was feeling about her losses. We discussed that her feelings were quite normal in the bereavement process. We discussed that I would be giving her some homework to do; some writing. I also suggested she spend more time outside her home, walking the paths of her farmland getting some exercise. I recommended she get a pet for a companion, perhaps a Labrador retriever.

 "They make excellent companion dogs." I stated with authority.

I knew a lot about Labs and recommend them often. I had one at home. I also knew about a kennel called Canine Helpers, an organization that specifically trained dogs to help the disabled and trained companion dogs as well. I gave Elsie the contact information and asked her to at least call and ask questions. She agreed.

Before I ended the first session, I asked perhaps the most important question for her. "Elsie, would you tell me about your spiritual condition. How are you feeling spiritually?" I paused giving her a minute.

I continued, "Spiritual healing is just as important as physical and mental healing."

Elsie remained silent. She looked down at her hands in her lap and fidgeted. I asked if she was a praying woman and suggested, if she was and was not praying like she may have done in the past, that she start praying more often.

Elsie looked up and whispered, "My husband and I were very active in our community church, Vic. Murdock was an elder in the church." She sniffled, raising her hankie to her nose, "I was a Sunday school teacher. We are a Christian family—even Jared was a believer—and we have been for many years."

I listened intently. I have always felt a higher power (many call that power God or Jesus Christ) a significant part of recovery and all important in the process of mending a broken heart or wounded soul.

Elsie continued, "My family has been devout Baptists for over four generations. I love the Lord, Vic. I just have had so much to adjust to in the last year, and with the loss of Jared and Gavin...," she paused looking directly into my eyes, "I have lost sight of what is important to me. Praying is one of those things."

And so it was that Elsie left my counseling office that day feeling some relief from the negative feelings, but there was much more left to do. I recall sending her home with a writing assignment that first day. I wanted her to write a letter saying goodbye to Jared. I specifically suggested she write it expressing her inner most feelings rather than what she was thinking. For example:

> *Dear Jared*
> *I feel...*
> *Signature*

Many therapists, including me, call this form of therapy, *expressive therapy*; it uses the act of writing and processing the written word as a therapeutic release of emotion. In Elsie's situation expressive therapy suggested that writing her feelings will gradually ease her pain of guilt, loss, and sadness.

Months went by. I was able to meet with Elsie each week at the clinic. She shared her letters with me, letters written to Jared, Gavin, God, herself and to me. They contained some very private and amazing disclosures. During each face-to-face counseling session, we discussed the feelings she had expressed in each of the letters. She opened-up and had a lot to say. I said very little. I mostly listened. She was on the mend.

Her very first letter she wrote to her son. In it, she referred to the time Jared was unable to come home from the war zone in Iraq when his father unexpectedly took a turn for the worse, extremely ill with terminal pancreatic cancer. Jared had been contacted in Iraq, but by the time he was informed and received new orders to go home to be with his father, it was too late. Gavin Murdock had already passed away, and Jared Murdock was still sitting in the air base terminal many thousands of miles away from his home, waiting for his flight out, still wearing his battle camouflage fatigues with the dust of the desert still on his boots from battle.

The description of Jared's anger and anguish Elsie described in her postmortem letter to Jared was heart wrenching. I had heard some of his story in counseling sessions but nothing like this, from the heart of a mother.

I tilted my head tilted backward, closing my eyes, as she read. I can only imagine the cavernous pain that must have pierce Jared's heart the moment he heard his father had died. Can anyone envision the tormenting thought that he never made it back to the States in time to be by his father's side when he needed him most?

Elsie did an amazing job putting into words her feelings in her letter to Jared. She wrote a forgiving message to her son, trying to explain how only now she is beginning to realize the emotional pain he had to be enduring prior to him taking his life. She read from her letter, "And now I am sitting here, angry at life some days, struggling to find the meaning of life other days. I search to make sense of it all. I feel I have lost my direction in life, son. Without you and your father I feel abandoned and left behind. I miss you and your dad, wondering what I could have done differently to prevent you from destroying your own precious life. And I mourn."

Elsie tried to control herself as she read her handwritten letter, but tears dripped onto the pages in her lap. The ink smeared slightly as she tried to dry the surface.

After a few moments, she sniffled and continued, "I ask your forgiveness, my dear Jared, for not being there for you in your time of trouble. If only I would have known more about your troubled thinking, I would have done anything in the world to save you—even giving up my own life. Good-bye, good boy. May the Lord bless and keep you in His loving and forgiving arms forever and ever! Love, Mom."

Elsie broke down, burrowed into her chair.

This was an unbelievable moment for me. I felt fortunate to bear witness to a huge breakthrough. The sense of the released burden Elsi had been carrying filled the room. I felt, saw, and heard the relief in Elsie's every word. This was truly an amazing story of triumph and perseverance.

Elsie appeared weak and exhausted; I offered her water. She took a sip. She had no more word. I had none, either. We just sat quietly for a long time.

As time passed, we completed our counseling sessions. Nevertheless, I would check up on Elsie Murdock from time to time by phone, a follow-up to find out how she was getting along. In fact, on one occasion, I drove out to the Murdock Farm not too far from our clinic just outside the city. And wouldn't you know it, who do you think ran up to greet me at the staircase to the porch—a yellow Labrador retriever!

CHAPTER 6

# Hard Time Prison

His face contorted and red and his body stiffened as he revisited battlefield scenes in his mind, Danny Barnes began to speak in group: "…opiate addict, parolee fresh out of prison for aggravated assault, nearly killed a guy with my 'K-BAR' in a bar fight. I was high on heroin—thought I was in the 'Nam' Delta Company 1968… done 8 years hard time, Sing Sing Prison, New York."

He shared these gut-level words, starring directly at me, his eyes burning a path into my heart. "…64-year-old former 1st Lieutenant Danny Barnes, US Marine Corp, Infantry Weapons Officer. I served in Vietnam during the Tet Offensive."

"In prison," he paused, clearing his throat, "I discovered a grotesque life— prison drug dealers, power-tripping guards, gang-banging psychopaths, jailhouse snitches, and hustling by any means necessary." He paused again and looked up at the ceiling, rubbing his face with his hands.

I had observed for several weeks now how deeply entrenched this warrior's anger and rage were, ever since his haunting war experience in the battle of Hue in 1968. I could see and feel his desperate need to tell his story to a group of veterans who have already walked his talk.

He began again, looking around group room 2. "Prisons work differently in different states. It can be challenging to know what exactly you need to do when a friend or family member is incarcerated. Sing Sing contains both male and female offenders. The levels of custody at the Sing Sing encompass minimum security all the way to maximum and death row. The Sing Sing Correctional Facility believes that the success of inmates starts while they are in prison. From day one, offenders are preparing for their release back into society. They begin assessments that help the Warden establish a plan for the inmate. Education, treatment, and life skills are all evaluated. These evaluations help staff to set goals for recovery, rehabilitation, and skill development so that an inmate will have the tools needed to lead a successful, crime-free life once they return to society." Danny took a sip from the silver drink container he had brought to group.

Indeed, research has proven that inmates who have a strong support system are more likely to be rehabilitated. The Correctional Facilities encourage positive friends and family who are law abiding to keep in contact with inmates while they are incarcerated.

Danny began again, looking around the room, "For those of you who plan on spending some time upstate, visitation times and days depended on the facility where an inmate is housed. Before you can schedule a visit, however, you will need to be on the approved visitor list. You can get on this list by having an inmate send you a visitor application or by filling out a visitor application. Approval may take 21 to 45 days as you will need to pass a background check."

Danny had a toothy grin, but it was contagious. The group smiled and laughed.

Danny continued to share, "When inmates are close to being released, they will be given a release day and made aware of the rules of release. Although an inmate receives basic needs from the Sing Sing Correctional Facility, they may need additional items. Within every prison, there is a store specifically for inmates called the commissary. The commissary allows inmates to purchase certain basic items. If inmates want to purchase something from commissary, they need to have money on their account. There are several ways you can put money on an inmates commissary account.

Danny hesitated, looked at me with a taut face, and asked, "Vic, may I continue? I would like to share why I'm really here in group. Sing Sing was just a bump in my road. I learned why I fought for my freedom."

I gestured with a thumbs up.

He then began to speak with an obvious lower tone and seriousness. "The Tet Offensive in 1968 was a series of North Vietnamese attacks on more than 100 cities and outposts in South Vietnam, I know firsthand because I was there," he said emphatically with the authority of an Infantry Weapons Officer. "As I understood it, the offensive was an attempt to stir-up rebellion among the

South Vietnamese population and encourage the United States to scale back its involvement in the Vietnam War. Though U.S. and South Vietnamese forces managed to hold off the attacks, news coverage of the massive offensive shocked the American public and eroded support for the war effort. Despite heavy casualties, North Vietnam achieved a strategic victory with the Tet Offensive, as the attacks marked a turning point in the Vietnam War and the beginning of the slow, painful American withdrawal from the region. Later, I found out that as the celebration of the lunar new year, the Tet holiday is the most important holiday on the Vietnamese calendar. In previous years, the holiday had been the occasion for an informal truce in the Vietnam War between South Vietnam and North Vietnam."

"In early 1968, however," barreling forward with his narrative, he shared, "we learned the North Vietnamese military chose January 31 as the occasion for an offensive of surprise attacks aimed at breaking the stalemate in Vietnam. In coordination with North Vietnamese President Ho Chi Minh, the military brass believed that the attacks would cause Army of the Republic of Vietnam forces to collapse and stir-up discontent and rebellion among the South Vietnamese people. Further, Charlie believed the alliance between South Vietnam and the United States was unstable and hoped the offensive would drive the final wedge between them and convince American leaders to give up their defense of South Vietnam."

Danny Barnes continued, pulling from his clearly etched-in-eternity memory, "I recall on Jan. 31, 1968, communist forces had taken control of Hue, the third largest city in South Vietnam. U.S. forces began their counterassault at daybreak as Delta Company, my unit, moved quietly through the maze-like alleyways and courtyards of the ancient city. The oldest part of Hue, a fortification that was built to protect the city when it served as the imperial capital of Vietnam, if I remember my history correctly."

Clearly, Barnes remembered what he saw as if it happened yesterday. Then, he spit out of his contorted mouth and spluttered angrily, "It was just sheer ruin: burned out automobiles and bodies on the road. The stench of death was there all the time." He twisted in his seat, red in the face, beads of sweat rolling down his brow, and paused.

Danny continued to speak after a minute, more in control, "By mid-afternoon, our company commander and the remaining uninjured men regrouped at Dong Ba Tower. This was one of the city's tallest structures. The tower was the main military objective for our U.S. forces as it would give us a strategic vantage point within the city. The strategy was straightforward: Charge the tower, kill the remaining enemy soldiers, and hold it. It turns out the reality would be far less easy. North Vietnamese army soldiers crouched in sniper foxholes within the tower and hid behind rubble to shoot U.S. Marines. On that morning of February 16, my rifle squad of 13 men launched their final assault on the Dong Ba Tower, nicknamed *the hill* because it looked like a pile of rubble after the initial combat."

Barnes described how his rifle squad fought the communist forces throughout the morning and by midday had reclaimed the tower. By the end of the fight to take Dong Ba Tower, out of the three rifle squads in his rifle platoon, six Marines were dead (two were his battle buddies) and several others injured. The rifle squad pulled 27 enemy bodies from the rubble after they consolidated their positions on the tower. By nightfall, the U.S. Marines were in control of *the hill.*

Danny paused for breath for a moment. Then, he spoke more softly, his head bobbing as he looked at the faces of the other vets around the room, "I might mention here—many of you already know this—troops familiar with fighting in dense jungles could be disoriented by combat in tightly packed streets. Sounds ricocheted off walls, adding to the confusion of urban combat. Crumbled buildings and blind corners made perfect sniper nests and ambush points. It was crazy chaos, man."

He stopped and rubbed his eyes with the palms of his hands, Then, he resumed, "Then, what I thought was the turning point of the war, there was a particularly bold attack on the U.S. Embassy in Saigon, a Viet Cong platoon got inside the complex's courtyard before U.S. forces destroyed it."

The fearless attack on the U.S. Embassy, and its initial success, stunned American and international observers, who saw images of the carnage broadcast on television as it occurred. The North had succeeded in achieving surprise, but Northern forces were spread too thin in the ambitious offensive. So, U.S. and South Vietnam forces managed to successfully counter most of the attacks. We inflicted heavy Viet Cong losses.

Particularly intense fighting took place in the city of Hue, located on the Perfume River some 50 miles south of the border between North and South Vietnam, The Battle of Hue would rage for more than three weeks after

Viet Cong forces burst into the city on January 31, easily overwhelming the government forces there and taking control of the city's ancient citadel.

Early in their occupation of Hue, Viet Cong soldiers conducted house-to-house searches, arresting civil servants, religious leaders, teachers, and other civilians connected with American forces or with the South Vietnamese regime. They executed these so-called counterrevolutionaries and buried their bodies in mass graves.

U.S. forces discovered evidence of the massacre after they regained control of the city on February 26. In addition to more than 2,800 bodies, another 3,000 residents were missing, and the occupying forces had destroyed many of the city's grand temples, palaces and other monuments.

The toughest fighting in Hue occurred at the ancient citadel, which the North Vietnamese struggled fiercely to hold against our superior firepower. In scenes of carnage recorded on film by numerous television crews on the scene, nearly 150 U.S. Marines were killed in the Battle of Hue, along with some 400 South Vietnamese troops.

Danny Barnes related this history with his own detail and personal emotions. He kept talking to me and the other 11 combat veterans in group room # 2 as if needing to download and glance over toward me as if looking for reassurance it was alright to continue to talk.

"Reports kept coming into our positions: on the North Vietnamese side, an estimated 5,000 soldiers were killed, most of them hit by American air and artillery strikes. What I saw was probably the most intense ground fighting on a sustained basis over several days of any other period during the war. We never seemed to know where the enemy was coming from, or in which direction even. We all know the outcome… yes?"

Danny stopped talking and looked across the room at me. "Well, Vic, that's it for me. Sorry I talked so long, just kept going! Sorry, guys and you, ladies." Everyone in the room waved arm motions of acceptance and understanding, a couple of fist-bumps and Oorahs.

Lieutenant Danny Barnes sat forward in his chair, steady, shirt soaked through around the arm pits and collar. His face faded reddish around the cheeks and tips of his ears. The blue tie-dye shirt sticking to his skin showed the outline of a muscular chiseled chest with dark long curly hairs bursting upward from the open shirt collar just under his chin. Quiet calmness now settled over the room.

Lieutenant Barnes is a heroin addict, a drug addiction he picked up overseas in theater. In America, the phrase, *opioid crisis,* has quickly made its way into my consciousness in the past few years —especially fentanyl. There has been a constant thread weaving through news stories, political speeches, and election campaign debates around what to do about the epidemic that's consuming whole communities, including the military and veteran population. It is currently reported that opioids account for more than two-thirds of deaths from drug overdoses and that number is only rising, with synthetic opioids, like fentanyl, being the driving force.

Medications have been the gold standard for treating opioid use disorder, but behavioral interventions can improve treatment for opioid addiction and address the comorbid conditions that go along with it. Fentanyl is a synthetic opioid pain reliever. It is many times more powerful than other opioids and is approved for treating severe pain, typically advanced cancer pain. Illegally made and distributed fentanyl has been on the rise in several states. Fentanyl, including illicitly manufactured fentanyl, may be mixed with heroin, cocaine, or other illicit drugs, increasing their potential lethality. Some factors increase a person's risk of opioid addiction even before they start taking these drugs — legally or otherwise. A person is at increased risk of opioid addiction if he or she:

- is a younger age, specifically the early 20s;
- is living in stressful circumstances, including being unemployed or living below the poverty line;
- has a personal or family history of substance abuse;
- has a history of problems with work, family and/or friends;
- has had legal problems in the past, including jail time;
- is in regular contact with high-risk people or high-risk environments where there's drug use;
- has struggled with severe depression or anxiety;
- tends to engage in risk-taking or thrill-seeking behavior; and/or
- uses tobacco heavily.

Several additional factors—genetic, psychological, and environmental—play a role in addiction, which can happen quickly or after many years of opioid use. Anyone who takes opioids is at risk of becoming addicted, regardless of age, social status, or ethnic background.

Common signs of opioid addiction include

- regularly taking an opioid in a way not intended by the doctor who prescribed it, including taking more than the prescribed dose or taking the drug for the way it makes a person feel;

- taking opioids "just in case," even when not in pain;

- mood changes, including excessive swings from elation to hostility;

- changes in sleep patterns;

- borrowing medication from other people or "losing" medications so that more prescriptions must be written;

- seeking the same prescription from multiple doctors, in order to have a "backup" supply;

- poor decision-making, including putting himself or herself and others in danger;

- if someone you love is addicted to opioids, you're also likely to experience changes in your thoughts and behaviors.

Friends and family of addicts may find themselves

- worrying about the addict's drug use, ranging from persistent anxiety to full-blown fear that their friend or loved one is going to die;

- lying or making excuses for the addict's behavior;

- withdrawing from the addict to avoid mood swings and confrontations; and/or

- thinking about or acting on the urge to call the police when the addict uses drugs or uses illegal means to obtain them.

It's common—and entirely human—to avoid addressing concerns for fear that relationship or family will fall apart. Friends and family may convince themselves that they'd know it was time for action if their loved one's addiction was truly serious. Even doctors may overlook common signs of opioid abuse, assessing the people they treat through the lens of "knowing them" versus an objective assessment of opioid-related problems.

# CHAPTER 7

# Family Dynamics

I first talked to Chad Williams over the phone at our clinic. His voice was raspy but discernable. I listened actively and with a clear focus.

Chad's story is about a family's determination and courageous attempt to rescue their loved one. The veteran's wife had called the clinic. "I may have to hang the phone up quickly. My husband is not himself," she whispered, sounding jittery and upset. "I don't know him anymore. I am afraid for my safety at times when he drinks too much, but I love the man. He never was a drinker, but now I don't know what to think. I can't leave him. He says he wants to hurt himself. He is so angry. What can I do?" She pleaded for help.

"You already have taken the important first step in helping your husband: You called us for help. Good work. It must have been very difficult," I responded.

She audibly sighed, seemingly with relief but also caution. "I am afraid of what he would do if he knew I made this call tonight; he loses his temper a lot lately. It has taken me several months to build up the courage to call for help. I opened this letter to my husband we received from Veteran Affairs months ago telling us about the signs of suicide to look for. My son also read it and kept asking me to make the call for his dad's sake—for our sake. I have the letter right here. but we don't go to the VA. My husband feels it is a sign of weakness if he goes in so we asked our private doctor. He gave us your phone number to call if we needed help outside of the VA. My husband needs help right now. He has over half of these danger signs listed in the letter it says here. I don't know which way to turn."

"What is your name?" I calmly inquired. There was silence for a moment. She appeared to be reluctant to give me her name. I waited.

Then, she spoke, "Elaine."

"Elaine, you have made the right decision to call me—a very good decision. Now, I need to ask you a few questions and get some additional information so that we can take good care of your veteran. Does he have a weapon?" I asked.

"I don't think so; I haven't seen one around the house," she replied.

"Has he hurt himself or anyone else?" I continued.

"No, but I'm not sure about the pills he takes for sleeping; he has them in his room. He wakes up in the middle of the night sometimes screaming words I don't understand and his legs flying around under the sheets. It scares me," the vet's wife sniffled into the receiver.

"Elaine, has your husband ever attempted suicide?"

She sounded somewhat surprised by the question. "Him? No way!" She sounded slightly amused. "He is Mr. Tough Guy, a real survivor, a good soldier, too. He has been decorated for combat—some commendations, I think, but never talks much about them or his time over there."

She continued sparingly, "He doesn't think that way, or at least he didn't use to. I am not sure anymore what he is thinking. He has really changed since his deployment home. It is hard for us. He won't go in for help."

"Your husband's condition is treatable, Elaine, and his mental health is not a sign of weakness by any means. He is not alone in this struggle. Many families are going through what you are experiencing right now. And I will tell you, Elaine, from my years of firsthand experience, many families in similar circumstances are restored and their veterans recover. Trust me on this. I am not saying that just to make you feel better. That is the truth. A great number of troops come home from Iraq and Afghanistan and as far back as Vietnam are still suffering and struggling in psychological confusion. I will help you get him in for help, okay?"

"It's so hard to believe he is having so much trouble this long after he was over there. We have got to do something," she said with questioning sadness in her tone.

"What is your husband's name?"

"Chad Williams." She responded quickly. "Sergeant Chad Williams, United States Army."

"What is his date of birth?"

"June 23, 1979." Again, she answered with a quick response as if she wanted the conversation to move along or end. I am not sure which.

"What is your address?" I continued.

"Wait a minute! I don't want you calling in the police! Hold on here! Chad doesn't know I called you. You are going to get me into real trouble here." Her voice swelled, and she sounded annoyed.

"Elaine, hold on, I am not calling the police or an ambulance unless you or your husband wants an emergency rescue. If there are any signs he has taken those pills or hurt himself in anyway, we will need to call for an ambulance. We need to check it out right now. If he hasn't, we will try and talk to him, all right?" I said, retreating a bit.

This is a real conversation and a story of hope, strength and courage. You will witness how Elaine and her son pulled together as a family during this difficult time. I guided Elaine to talk to her wounded suicidal warrior suffering with unrelenting symptoms of suicidal thought and to learn how to stay connected and keep lines of communication open—and especially to take suicidal ideation seriously.

A significant other of a suicidal veteran generally lives under immense pressure. Elaine told me, "Most of the time I try to be especially careful about my speech and behavior toward my husband and try to do whatever I can to minimize the stresses in his life to avoid making him angry and threatening to kill himself. I hate when he says that. I don't know when to believe him or not."

Case in point, Elaine found herself carefully monitoring not only her own actions, but also those of her son. "We can't upset your father, "she often told her son.

She had tried to make life easier for her husband by not pressuring him to attend certain social and family get-togethers. At first, she had been willing to go alone. Eventually, however, she stopped going out at all and became reclusive, like her wounded warrior. Elaine was beginning to realize just how damaging her isolation had been to her own mental health.

Even after a heightened suicidal threat has subsided and a vet appears calmer and more elevated in mood, a partner needs to be aware that suicide can occur at any time. Sometimes, the veteran seems improved, but it may be because of the result of an inner decision to commit suicide at some future time and thereby terminate what he or she perceives as an intolerably painful and hopeless way of life. My research indicates 75 percent of people who commit suicide hint that they plan to do so. Often, the veteran might say things like "You would be better off without me here" or start giving away his or her possessions. Other signs of suicidal depression include withdrawing from normal family activities.

A proper response is to validate the veteran's concerns. Even if the problems may not seem big to others, they are very real to the vet in crisis. I explained to Elaine how it would help to show compassion for the pain Chad was experiencing, to tell him how much she cared. Reinforcing a shared connection is the first step to preventing a vet's suicide.

"Elaine, I sincerely suggest to you that the important essentials in helping to rescue your husband are open channels of communication," guiding her intervention strategy by suggesting that she "say what you must say and do what you must do to keep the relationship between you and Chad undamaged, however shaky it may be. In your situation, Elaine, the conversation with Chad will be through direct dialogue face-to-face or through his closed door, right?"

"Yes, but I don't know if he will open the bedroom door and come out of his room to talk to me. He is sleeping in the spare bedroom and sometimes doesn't come out for days," she replied in a nervous and agitated manner.

"Mrs. Williams, I believe the best thing to do in your situation, and right now, because he may have taken those pills already, would be a face-to-face conversation with him asking him to come to the phone and telling him that a counselor, a veteran, would like to speak with him. If he asks who made the phone call, tell him the truth that you called the clinic because you love him and are concerned about him and how he is acting right now. Don't mention his suicidal threats. Can you try to do that, Elaine?"

Once again there was an awkward silence.

"You seem upset, Elaine, and understandably so. This is a tough situation you are in, but you can do this. I know you can do this. You have already shown me your courage and determination to help Chad. So, please talk to me. If you do not understand what I am suggesting for you to do, tell me, okay?"

I heard her breathing on the line. I remained silent for a minute hoping and praying she would follow through and persuade her husband to come out of his room and come to the phone. She said nothing. I could almost hear her mind bustling as I continued in a controlled voice, "I can always send a rescue team out to help you if you can't do this. But I can't ignore your plea for help. In fact, Elaine, your husband is also crying out for help; these things I know."

"I am listening but not so sure I can do it," Elaine replied hesitantly.

"If you fear confronting him, talk to him through the door he is hiding behind. Is the door barricaded or locked from inside? "I asked.

"I don't really know. I stay away from him when he gets like this. I have heard him moving something around in there from time to time. Don't really know," she said.

At this point, I suggested again to Elaine that any conversation with her husband perhaps should not begin with reference to the fact that he was threatening to kill himself and was at the moment the center of his own distress and anxiety. Rather, the talk should begin by directing the conversation in a particular way toward a particular objective, such as getting Chad to safety. In this situation, the objective was to talk with me on the phone. The rescuer, in this case Elaine, may then state how she wants to be of service to her husband (in any way possible) and then ask him how he thinks he can be assisted in his obvious dilemma. If Chad draws back and refuses to respond or otherwise indicates hopelessness, Elaine must continue in offering a variety of conversational remarks in the hope of winning an acknowledgment, such as

- "Can I get you some food or something to drink?" or
- "Would you like me to bring you something to read?"

In this small way, she is engaging her husband in conversation. The part of the veteran's consciousness or psyche that desires to be rescued has begun to accept the possibility that a way out of this hopelessness can be found. The longer dialogue continues, the less the likelihood of a sudden desperate decision to harm himself and the greater the possibility of the eventual successful intervention.

"Elaine, are you ready to talk with your husband?" I coached.

I have to, don't I?" she responded uncertainly.

"No, you do not, but I highly recommend that I talk to him right now on the phone and get him the help he needs. And the only one who can get him to do that at this moment is you. Elaine. We need to do this right now. We don't know what his suicidal mind is thinking. We cannot hesitate to act at times like this. Suicidal ideation is very unpredictable. I will wait here on the phone while you go talk to Chad. I will wait as long as it takes. I won't hang up." I tried to reassure her.

"Wait a minute. I am going to put the phone down and go talk to him. He is upstairs ... wait a minute ... not sure about this. He is not going to like this ... What is your name?" she asked, understandably upset.

"Vic ... Vic Montgomery." I heard the receiver thump on a hard surface. Then silence.

I was sitting at my wooden oak desk in the clinic office. I put my head in my hands, elbows on the desk and massaged my temples with my forefingers round and round, pushing the tips into my hair line. *This was stressful.* I do that from time to time to relax. The minutes went ticking by on the clock on the wall. I waited. As I closed my eyes for a moment, I began to think about the situation Elaine was in and how I wished I was physically there to take over this intervention for her because I have the experience and training. It was obvious she was afraid of the outcome.

Then my thoughts shifted to Chad. My heart hurt for this warrior. Tears began to well up in my eyes. He is fighting to stay alive...once again, I reflected. What a hero! "We have to save this family," I said out loud.

My mind drifted... began thinking about some of my training ...*a search for an alternative to suicide begins when the veteran starts to speak of his or her pain. Elaine did not have the restricted view of her suicidal husband. She could suggest to him that living is worth trying and the loss of his platoon buddy in combat is a terrible blow, but the worth of those who die soldiers on in the lives and work of the survivors. Hope in the possibilities of the future is the most important concept for Elaine to put into words since her depressed veteran thinks narrowly only of a minuscule range of time in the here and now. If the vet identifies with the death of a war buddy, suggest the possibility of new relationships. As an appeal to the right of the person at risk, consider him or her not unlike other persons. Remind him that the suicide he proposes as a solution to this problem is, in a sense, unfair. If the veteran enforces a death sentence on himself for failing to save the life of his friend, then, by the application of simple justice, every veteran who fails to save a life should be subject to execution. Only the most delusional veteran will miss the obvious futility of that implication. To reintroduce a concept of self-worth to a combat veteran whose self-image is damaged, it's essential that offered promises be simple, within the sphere of realistic possibility, and consistent with the veteran's values. The self-punishing veteran perhaps can't believe he can ever again take responsibility or be dependable on account of some mistake or letdown from the past, even one that he could not have prevented. Veterans wrestle with self-blame and self-hatred. During battle, the pandemonium of war combined with physical and emotional stress can create frequent situations where even the most dedicated and accomplished combat warrior could easily have a lapse in judgment. When that mistake results in a loss of a buddy or part of his patrol, this warrior's self-blame can be so enormous as to produce rage at himself for the mistake he made. Others speak angrily to themselves for personal behavior they perceive as spineless and weak or needlessly vicious. The self-blaming warrior defines himself as a failure by reasonable criteria applied to anyone else he considers trustworthy and capable. An intervention should be aimed at countering the forces of self-contempt and their likely rundown in the elimination of the hated object, the failed self. This comes into play most often with veterans suffering from survivor guilt.*

The phone line was still silent. Twenty minutes had gone by since my last words with Elaine. I heard nothing in the background. The last thing in the world I want is a hang-up. Disconnections are such an empty feeling when they happen. And they happen quite often on the hotline when the fear is just too great for the caller on the other end, be they veteran or family member. The heartbreaking thing is help is only a matter of minutes away. Life and death lay in the balance. I read a news article recently that said the number of Afghanistan and Iraq combat troops and veterans who committed suicide had doubled from 2006 to 2007 and that "100,000 OEF/OIF vets have sought help for mental health issues, including 52,000 for post-traumatic stress disorder alone."

I couldn't help but think about the possibility that Elaine's husband might have had other means with which to take his life other than the pills she knew he had. Now I am second guessing myself, I thought. Maybe I should dispatch a rescue team, at least for a welfare check. Elaine has been away from the phone for a while now. I am getting concerned. Should I call 911? My mind began working overtime as thoughts raced through my mind.

Suddenly, I heard Elaine's keyed up voice loud and clear coming through my headset, "He is coming … he said he would talk to you …oh, he looks terrible—" she abruptly stopped talking as if someone else came into the room. Elaine was sobbing. The next moment, "Yeah, who's this?" a gruff, shaky voice demanded.

"Hello, Chad, this is Vic. Your wife and son are concerned about you, buddy. Your family love and care about you, Sergeant Williams. I am a vet, too, and a counselor. I can help you get through these tough times if you will let me, Chad. Have you hurt yourself in any way?

"Well…," he hesitated as if searching for the right words. "What's your name again?"

"Vic Montgomery, Chad. I work for a healthcare clinic not far from you. We have a vet's group that meets weekly that has combat vets just like you. I would like to invite you to come in and see me. How about today, Chad, say 2 this afternoon or would 3 o'clock be better?"

Chad was slow to respond. I heard him clear his pharynx. "My wife probably already told you I thought about hurting myself. I have been feeling down for a long time…don't know…sometimes things get crazy. My head won't shut down—too many memories; I still can't get a good night's sleep after all these years, Vic."

"Chad, have you thought of a plan to hurt yourself?" I inquired.

"Many times…," he paused. "Are you kidding me?" he shouted out suddenly straining his high-pitched voice. "For a long time…" he hesitated, "I have a good supply of my sleeping pills I am prescribed. Maybe I shouldn't be telling you this. I thought about jumping in my car and ending it all the other day. There is a very nice cliff at the end of our street that would be perfect. And my wife would get some insurance to boot—money is tight around here. I haven't been able to keep a steady job for years since getting back from Afghanistan. I get angry and upset easily. It got ugly over there, thinking you're going to die every day. Well, it's tough to live with, man. You got to be there to feel it. "

I interrupted him to ask, "Chad, are you seeing a VA doctor about these things?"

"Hell, no. I went to a civilian doc for my trouble sleeping. He is the one who gives me the pills. I don't want the VA to know any of this," he admitted.

"Chad, listen to me. It takes the courage of a warrior to ask for help. I am proud of you for talking to me tonight. This alone takes backbone. I would like to get some help for you, buddy. From the things you have shared with me just now and the few concerns Elaine told me, I can see why you are having a tough time of it."

I paused. Chad said nothing.

"I would like you to do something for me. Would you please temporarily give all your pills, car keys, any alcohol or drugs you have and anything else that may put you into harm's way right now, please give them over to your wife to hold on to. Can you do that?" I asked in a beseeching manner.

Still no sound from Chad.

"Chad, talk to me. I want to help you buddy. I've got your six, man. But the only way I can help you is if you cooperate with me and allow me to make sure you and your family are safe."

"I'm listening," the broken veteran muttered but was slow to respond further. I listened and waited for more from him before I continued.

"What do you mean you can help me? What kind of help?"

"Chad, there are several options that I can provide for you, but before we discuss those options, would you please give those items I previously discussed over to your wife right now just to hold for you? I will wait on the line, and when that is done, I will explain to you what the next step is to getting you support. Can you do that?" I waited for a response. Nothing. Not even an utterance or the noise of his breath although I was certain he hadn't hung up.

"Listen to me, buddy. I understand how difficult it is for you to ask for help. Many combat warriors have thick skin and a tough constitution. You are a seasoned warrior and have learned in combat to suck it up and stuff your feelings. Your wife was bragging earlier about how you were a tough guy, a good soldier, and decorated. Ooh-rah!" I empathized, accentuating the age-old Marine war cry.

Suddenly, there came a faint "Oorah" back at me over the receiver. It made me smile to hear him say that.

"So, what I propose Chad is for you to come into my clinic office and meet with me for a face-to-face appointment, as soon as possible, say tomorrow morning at 10 a.m., and attend one of our veterans' groups tomorrow evening at 6 o'clock in group room #2. Will you commit to this Chad?" I waited. There was silence.

"Hear me on this, Chad. Many combat veterans have finally come to realize, especially with the help and encouragement of their battle buddies, families, and other loved ones, that haunting nightmares, flashbacks, and depression finally begin to take their tolls. We can help you work through these nightmares, traumatic combat memories, and sleepless nights. We can, and we will, soldier," I said assertively.

Chad said, "OK! I will be there. Thank you for listening to me, Vic. Let's get this thing going, bro."

## Steps to Prevent a Veteran's Suicide

- Confront the veteran with the probability he has been planning suicide and has lethal means at hand. Request that he voluntarily turn over his guns, car keys, knives, beer and liquor and cache of pills to a trusted relative or friend. Encourage him to communicate and confide his fantasy of carrying out his death. Encourage the vet to talk.

- Remove lethal means and opportunity from the veteran or vice versa at the earliest possible opening

- Ask questions to find a reason for him/her to live, feeding the warrior's heart and soul with winning encouragement and affirmations. When the veteran is stabilized, finding some glimmer of "hope of help" diminishes the suicide risk.

Get the veteran to safety is by connecting the veteran to supporting Veteran Resources Appendix B at the end of this book or local emergency services in the community or a VA Medical Center wherever he or she lives. The federal government, Congress, has mandated a follow-up protocol for all suicide and crisis calls: they are to be referred for a private, confidential consultation with a well-trained, professional suicide prevention coordinator at one of the more than 153 VA Medical Centers throughout the United States.

# CHAPTER 8

# Sexual Assault

As I approached the reception desk in the clinic waiting room to pick up the yellow file folder for my next appointment, I noticed a set of piercing green eyes staring at me from across the room. She was the only female in the room so I decided this must be my next appointment: Alice Anderson.

I opened the file folder, glancing at the information page, paused only for a moment, then flipped the cover closed, and, turning on my heel, walked over to where Alice was sitting. As I approached her, I extended my hand, saying, "Hello, I am Vic Montgomery. Are you Alice Anderson for a 2 o'clock with me?"

She squeezed my hand, nodded, and said yes in a raspy tone. Her beautiful but aging face showed signs of wear and tear in places. Her lips were lined with a deep red lipstick. Alice wore tight, faded blue jeans with a dark blue, long sleeve shirt and collar revealing a colorful beaded neckless laying against her rounded breast line. She sat straight up in her chair without a moment of hesitation when I approached her, her green eyes continuing to gleam. Alice had turned into a hard lady. learning to shoulder the burdens she was carrying for all these years.

I invited the veteran to walk with me to my office. Nurse Alice sat down; I offered her something to drink. She took coffee. I pulled a chair from next to my desk and placed it in front of her knees to be close and supportive—and focused. The Kleenex was on a small table to the right of her. We began with small talk and getting to know each other. Then, after a short time, having gathered assessment information and shared my professional qualifications and experience, we really began to talk.

This 33-year-old military nurse veteran appeared worn out and deeply saddened. In fact, she looked like she was ready to explode. I began to learn she had turned in to a heroin addict and cutter ever since she was raped while in the military war zone.

I clearly remember thinking, *in many cases, veterans' emotions are raw and untested. Questions many times run through their minds whether the counselor will understand them, Will the counselor judge them?* The internal pain is just too much and the fear of sharing a personal tragedy, their stories, with anyone appears to be a gigantic feat. Alice's overwhelming feeling of isolation was so apparent and powerful I felt the enormity of the moment.

"Take as much time as you need," I gently responded to her silent cry for help. She began to weep.

As I handed her the Kleenex box, I thought about the trauma she must have endured for all these years; sexual trauma is another form of trauma that can lead to psychological complications and suicide ideation. I also knew from experience compounding the issue that sexual aggressors are often military comrades, and once a victim of sexual assault is deemed physically safe, the trauma is not over. Sexual trauma's mental health impact is a serious problem for veterans coming home from war zones. I recall how The National Online Resource Center on Violence Against Women explained to me some years ago the different responses victims have to sexual trauma as psychological consequences of sexual trauma, responses that are diverse and highly individualized. There is no one response that is experienced by all survivors (Yuan et al., 2009).

Alice continued crying quietly for several minutes before she began to speak again. It seemed like an eternity before she said another word.

"It is hard for people outside the war zone to understand how living in high stress, primitive conditions can affect your ability to make decisions," she declared, her voice quivering. "I didn't report the sexual harassment and attack immediately because I felt an obligation to continue the mission and not burden others." She explained that she also wondered how the mostly male upper command would perceive the report. "What would it do to my career and promotions? The Army was my life," she shared, still questioning her judgment.

Alice's story revealed the secrecy and moral burden of sexual trauma in the United States military. This honorable and dedicated military nurse perceived she was at the end of all possible hope for relief from the psychological demons that haunted her. Her life seemed to be over, and she saw no way out. It took this once confident veteran nurse several months to call our clinic after she was honorably discharged and separated from the Army.

Suddenly, Alice reached out and grabbed my hand pulling it toward her. She was shaking. I felt her bony hand trembling. She was inches in front of my face, green eyes staring directly into mine. Tears emanating from the corners of her eyes.

She began whispering; "Vic, I trust you with what I am about to tell you. Is this private?"

"Yes, it is, Mrs. Anderson, unless I determine you are going to harm yourself or others. Do you feel safe right now? Are you going to continue cutting yourself?"

"I will try to stop the cutting and using if you will help me."

"I will enroll you tonight."

She continued to speak, "I was sexually and emotionally abused, harassed, and raped by a fellow Army National Guard soldier while on duty in Iraq. When I deployed home, I felt I could not share this information with my family or anyone else, for that matter. I felt disconnected from my family. I began to isolate myself and am pretty much a loner today. I feel I have lost everything… my dignity and honor. And so, I decided to leave the service after eight years; I couldn't continue wearing the uniform. I felt dirty. I was and still am angry— and disgusted at myself. I just can't find anything to be happy about. I don't smile, Vic. I always had a smile on my face. It's like it is painted over with a brushstroke, a blank face, nothing there. I look in the mirror in the morning and don't know who I am anymore. I'm ugly. I was a happy person, Vic. Now I am hooked on drugs!" She began to cry.

"Take your time; you are safe here. I will help you." I tried to reassure her. "I am listening to every word you are sharing, Alice. I really care about what you are going through right now. I am so glad you came in to see me today. I will see to it that you get the help you need. Okay?" I was speaking from my heart.

I tried to encourage her. She made no response. I could hear her labored breathing as she continued, "I had a lot of friends. I enjoyed being around people. I have no desire to have a relationship. He hurt me, Vic. I hurt all over. I will never be the same again. What's the use of living? I have nothing to look forward to but this same miserable life I live day in and day out. I go to work and come home and sit like a zombie. I have difficulty sleeping many nights."

Alice shared with me how she felt her life was slowly fading away. It had been several years since the horrid experience. She told me how she was having continuing nightmares and flashbacks bringing back the memory of the attack and the distorted face of the unshaven rapist, an assumed American comrade-in-arms in the war zone of Iraq. She described the smell of his breath as "raunchy, filled with the rancid odor of alcohol and cigarettes." She paused for a moment as if to collect her thoughts and control her emotions.

She took some deep breaths. I remained silent and listened for more of her story but was ready to jump in and offer her kindhearted support.

Alice recalled, "The attacker was so angry he could not hold an erection or penetrate me, so he used his fingers, viciously saying, 'You like that, huh? You want more, sweetie pie?' as he pinned me down with his forearm pushing against my throat. I remember closing my eyes to escape; I went numb. Then, he was gone. Vic, I have never shared this with anyone, let alone a man. I don't know why I am saying this now, to you. I feel ashamed and embarrassed beyond belief." She paused. "I feel like running away! I am having a hard time holding this stuff in. I can't hold this inside any longer. I am going nuts." She took some Kleenex and blew her nose several times, wiping her eyes.

"Alice, you are doing the right thing coming to me today. I can help you get through this. May I ask you a few questions so I can give you the help you need and deserve?"

I wanted to move this intense, graphic conversation to another topic and ease the emotion that was building up the more she talked about the event, understandably so. *My word...what a burden to carry around for so long,* I thought. My experience and therapeutic training suggest that Alice's story needs to be told in a way that transfers the moral burden of the sexual attack in the war zone from the veteran to the community she served.

Storytelling is a very successful heart-to-heart resuscitation model for treatment. Sexual trauma survivors need to talk to active, sincere, and "in-the-present" listeners, people they can learn to trust and who encourage them to dive headlong into the stories with no hesitation and no holding back. Otherwise, the sexual trauma survivors might continuously repeat details of the event without experiencing the release of interrelated emotions, the precise memories of the past or the concept of consequence—all of which are indispensable in the recovery from a traumatic experience that may result in a therapeutic diagnosis of post-traumatic stress, depression, or anxiety disorders.

I cannot reiterate enough that these are all treatable conditions—treatable, in many cases, without a medication regiment or deeply invasive psychoanalysis. A professional counselor or other referral from your medical doctor is a wise decision; however, if fear exists to the extreme, causing the veteran not to seek help or treatment, then certainly a family member or good friend can be the trusted listener. Getting the right help is so vital.

The experiences Alice was going through were fragile. She needed to be handled with heart-to-heart caring and compassion. Alice needed to tell her story face-to-face with someone she could trust with the information, preferably a therapist familiar with combat trauma PTSD. The phone is not the place for this kind of conversation.

I would like to mention an important point and emphasize here that while trying to heal your emotional wounds for combat experiences initially, in the short term, your mind and body are struggling to cope with those traumatic experiences. But many times, your mind may still think it is in the danger zone again. And continue to think it is repeating that same trauma while continuing to struggle to make sense of what has just happened.

Here are some signs and symptoms of post-traumatic stress:

- Re-experiencing of the traumatic event(s)
- Stressful recollections
- Difficulty sleeping
- Flashbacks (feeling as if the sexual trauma is being experienced again)
- Nightmares (frequent recurrent images of the sexual trauma while asleep)
- Feeling disconnected from the world and the things happening in it
- Restricting emotions; "stuffing or self-medicating"
- Trouble remembering important parts of what happened during the trauma
- Shutting down (feeling emotionally and/or physically numb)

- Feeling anxious or fearful (as if back in that fearful place)
- Drawing inward or becoming emotionally numb
- Active avoidance of activities, places, thoughts, feelings, memories, people, or conversations related to or that bring the experience to mind
- Loss of interest
- Feeling detached from others (finding it hard to have loving feelings or experiencing any strong emotions or bonding relationships)

I began with some questions, "Alice, are you thinking about suicide?"

"I have thought about it, especially lately," she replied forlornly.

"What have you thought about?" I continued to probe.

"Cutting my wrists with a razor and going to sleep, hopefully escaping from these hopeless feelings. I am tired. Some days are worse than others," Alice responded despondently.

"Have you done anything to hurt yourself?" I asked.

"Oh, it seems I always hurt myself in one way or another. I cut myself on my legs when I am feeling badly. It kind of relieves the tension and takes the edge off. I got therapy when I was a teenager for cutting. I never have been one for using drugs or alcohol. My father was a drunk, and I swore I would never be like him. I hated my mother for living with him and putting up with all his abuse. So, I found I would get what relief I needed when I cut myself. The feeling is…well, I don't really want to go into it right now," she concluded abruptly.

Clinical studies indicate those who cut themselves do so to obtain the same euphoric level or release of emotional pressure as does the drug addict shooting up a syringe of heroin, the marijuana smoker smoking a joint, or the alcoholic polishing off a fifth of whiskey. These are all acts of self-medication and pleasure-seeking behavior. The serious and sad nature of these actions many times ends with an overdose and subsequently the death of the user. This is a matter of life and death at every turn (Tull, 2009).

"Alice, have you cut yourself today?" I begged for the answer.

"Well, some," she eked out.

I knew by that answer I had a high-risk-for-suicide vet with me.

"Alice, are you getting help for the cutting right now?"

"No! "She said emphatically.

"Alright, can I send you to the hospital to get someone to look at you?"

"No, Vic! Would you just stick to my head problem?"

"Ok! OK! Alice, I just wanted to be sure you are safe."

"Yes, Vic, I am safe. I am a nurse, remember?"

"Alice, we are about out time for today, I have another appointment coming up. How are you feeling? "

"Tired, Vic, but okay. I'm doing alright. Thanks for asking."

"Alice, I really do care about you and would like to invite you to join other vets I am working with in a group I run at 6 o'clock Tuesdays and Thursdays here at the clinic in group room # 2, just down the hall from my office."

"Bye for now, Vic, Thanks for listening. I'll think about it." She slowly strolled down the hall and out of the building.

As I watched Alice leave my office, I could not help but think about our private conversation and the fact she said she trusted me with her personal and sensitive information. I specifically remember thinking *what a breakthrough and so early in our treatment plan process.* This is huge in working with all clients! It also highly improves the recovery outcome from PTSD, sexual abuse, cutting and drug addiction for long term success (Tull, 2007).

I realized the moment Alice began sharing her fragile story that the diversity of her emotions and maladaptive behaviors pointed to post-traumatic stress symptoms such as depression, suicidal thoughts and attempts, and problem drug abuse. Many clinicians are now supporting diagnoses of Complex PTSD, which includes both PTSD and borderline personality disorder, as a way of better under-standing and treating sexual trauma survivors (Olenchek, 2008).

CHAPTER 9

# Relapse Prone

"Being an alcoholic is a lonely place to be. I can be in a room full of people and still feel all alone," shared veteran Jimmy Maxwell who served honorably in the U.S. Army's 1st Battalion of the 325th Airborne Infantry Regiment in Al -Fallujah, Iraq in 2003. The 34-year-old former Corporal, paratrooper, was relapsing prone. He had failed to complete four other alcohol and drug treatment programs over the last six years, but he keeps coming back for help. Recovery from alcohol addiction was challenging for him, like for many alcoholics, and he found himself relapsing, time after time. Before the light finally switches on, some never make it.

Several military media reports (Global Security, 2006), along with my medical records research, suggest that about 30% of veteran warriors who have returned home from combat have been diagnosed with signs of post-traumatic stress and/or traumatic brain injury. Substance abuse because of PTSD and TBI continues to be a growing concern.

It is crystal clear to me, after hearing the frantic, crisis-induced phone calls referred to our outpatient clinic from hundreds of family members, friends, and the vets themselves returning home from multiple tours of combat that the unrelenting direct orders to deploy a second, third and, in some cases, fourth tour to Iraq and Afghanistan is unconscionable. Numerous medical studies already indicate the incidents and severity of post-traumatic stress disorder and the onset of suicide ideation increased with each added tour.

An article on the Web site for the Pennsylvania-based NBC affiliate JAC-TV quotes Gordon Mathers (need citation) of the VA Medical Center as saying, "When they come back to the U.S., there's no on-and-off switch in their head just to say that it's all over. They don't miss the combat, but they miss booting up and being ready. The rush is like a drug addiction.

Conquering the addiction of a warrior's adrenaline rush and discovering how to recognize alcohol and substance dependency are important steps for a veteran's healing. I recollect a call where the caller blurted out these words almost immediately when I picked up the clinic's phone line: "I can't share anything with my family and friends. I don't want them to think I am a monster," the caller said, pausing and slurring his speech. "I began to love the smell of death and burned powder. The command ordered 'everyone needs to be eliminated.'"

The caller wanted to remain anonymous, but after I told him my name, "This is Vic," he told me his first one, Jimmy. However, he withheld his last name.

Jimmy's story was an emotional and painful one. He was a former combat Marine stationed in 2004 within the combat zone in the Iraqi city of Al-Fallujah, a large town 40 miles west of Baghdad. Fallujah was the most violence-prone area in Iraq, and since early April 2003, had experienced violent crowd control incidents, murders, and bombings.

As our phone call continued, Jimmy blurted out in fits and starts that he was only 33-years-old, his wife had left him for another man, and his best friend had committed suicide.

"I am listening," I said, not knowing what to expect next.

Jimmy continued, "I continually see bodies and their lifeless eyes in my dreams. I wake up soaked in sweat. I can't sleep. I began to love seeing the dead bodies of the enemy in front of me," he paused and sniffled. "I'm tired of hearing about the war. I don't know who I am anymore." He then lowered his gruff voice and mournfully said, "We came back home from Iraq, and after four months my Marine buddy blew his brains out." He paused. "I have a weapon. I can't get any rest. I have nothing to live for...no one left...my buddies are gone...and other friends...dead. I wrestle and toss and turn at night. I can't sleep, man. I see their lifeless eyes in my dreams." He paused again, sounding like he was taking a sip of something—the noise of a glass being rattled near the receiver.

After two tours in Al-Fallujah, Iraq, this veteran had lost his identity. Jimmy saw himself as a monster. He drank a fifth of whiskey a day to help suppress the inner turmoil. The combat veteran was discouraged and felt trapped. He was a suicidal, depressed warrior. He had lost his way; hence, the battle for personal survival was on. A cleansing of the mind often occurs through a careful process of bringing to the surface withdrawn, covered-up emotions and feelings in an effort to identify and relieve them. Jimmy needed help and guidance to learn how to release the combat adrenaline rush he still felt and to disown the addiction to that rush he had developed during his battle and bloodshed experiences.

I hesitated to say anything, because I felt as if this Marine needed to vent at that point, needed someone to listen to his obviously pent-up emotions. So, I just listened. I leaned forward, elbows on my desk. I looked up briefly at the clock on the wall. The evening was relatively calm for a Saturday. I heard Jimmy breathing into the receiver on the other end of the line. Then, he asked, "Hey! Are you there, or did I scare you away?" There was mockery in his tone.

"No, Jimmy. I am still here, buddy. I will not leave you. I am listening to you," I responded calmly, trying to defuse the emotional ranting and raving.

The warrior began speaking again, "I can still smell the decay of death. I will always remember. My mind repeats the same scenes. I am trapped in this insanity. It's over, man. It's over. I am going to hang up now. Shit, shit!"

I responded instinctively, "Wait, Marine, don't hang up. Give me another minute to talk with you. Oh, yes, you do have a reason to live, and I will tell you why! For one, I care, Jimmy. Semper Fi, brother! I care that you served our country with honor. Thank you for serving! Welcome home, Jimmy. Many people care whether you live or die. You have family who love you. They might not understand exactly what you are going through right now, but that can change if you will let me help you. I have your back, Marine. "Will you come into the clinic today and talk with me? Jimmy, listen to me, buddy, you are not alone in this battle. Let me help you right now."

There was a ghostly silence.

"Talk to me, Jimmy. Don't hangup, buddy!"

Click...dial tone. When he hung up the phone, my heart sank. A feeling of nausea came over me. My head dropped to the desk in fatigue and dejection. I couldn't help this Marine tonight, I thought. I began questioning my own abilities and conversation with the hurting Marine. What could I have said differently? I put the receiver back in the cradle while kicking the trash can. I looked distraughtly in the direction of the doorway.

I got up from my desk and took a walk down the hallway leading to the waiting room, my hands resting on the top of my head, fingers clasped and elbows in the air. I kicked open the outer door to the outside deck to get some fresh air. Thinking carefully, I continued to replay the conversation with Jimmy in my mind. At that moment, I was discouraged and saddened that I failed to bring a troubled warrior to safety. This is my job. It never gets routine or easy. We as clinicians must shake it off and get back on track for the next call or appointment.

A few minutes had passed on my walk outside of the building when I heard a shout coming down the corridor from a colleague, "Phone call, Vic. Someone asking to speak only to you by name."

I hurried back to my desk and picked up the line. It was Jimmy.

It is natural to push aside agonizing memories just as it is instinctive to avoid dangerous or unspeakable scenes in actuality. This natural tendency to cast out the stressful or the dreadful is especially well-defined in veterans, whose powers of resistance have been reduced by the long-continued strains of combat firefights, second and third tours, or other catastrophes of war incidents. Left to themselves, most vets would naturally strive to forget distressing memories and thoughts.

Jimmy was, however, very far from being left to himself. The natural tendency for hardened combat warriors is to repress feelings. In Jimmy's case, he was isolating and drinking heavily to numb the daily struggles and stressors of the day as well as the trauma of unfamiliar feelings of suicidal ideation.

I closed the door to my office, grabbed my telephone handset, and dug in for the call. "Jimmy, buddy, you had me worried. What's up? What's going on with you right now? Talk to me," I said, engaging him caringly.

Jimmy began to speak a bit calmer than before. I felt as if he were testing me to see if he could trust me with this unbelievably private, raw information. Possibly some fear hovered nearby.

"I can't talk to nobody about this stuff. How do you describe to family or friends or even a shrink what it was like to pull the trigger and watch your first kill crumple to the ground before you? How do I talk about the short bursts of bullets buzzing over my head and the fear and adrenaline rush inside of me? These people don't know anything. How can they understand what I feel inside my head and my heart? Man, this talking to you is no use. What can you do for me?" I continued to listen.

"I approached the Iraqi. He was just lying there, eyes and mouth wide open, just a kid. The thick blood was pooling around his head. " The warrior paused abruptly as if checking himself. I heard a bit of a frog in his throat.

"Jimmy, I am listening, and we can get you the help you need to work through these memories. And you aren't a monster, buddy. You were sent into battle. You are a Marine. Ooh-rah, you did what you had to do," I said with sensitivity.

"Are you a veteran, Vic?" Jimmy said inquisitively.

"Is that important to you, whether I am a veteran or not?" I asked.

"Yeah, kind of." Jimmy fell silent.

"What about my being a veteran would make you feel more comfortable?" I questioned.

"Oh, I don't know, just wondered, I guess. I feel like I can talk to you," he slurred.

"Jimmy, I want to get you to come in and see me at the clinic as soon as possible," I pleaded. "Would you agree to that so we can get you to where you are safe and out of harm's way. I would like to talk with you face-to-face…. Jimmy, you have a weapon, and that concerns me, buddy. You have already told me you want to end your life."

Jimmy uneasily interrupted, "When my wife and I were together, she worried. She couldn't understand why I repeatedly jumped out of bed in the middle of the night screaming war cries. I don't blame her for leaving me. I am some kind of monster." Jimmy slurred his words again. "But I miss her and can't take this being alone any longer, day in and day out. I feel hopeless, man, just sitting and staring out the window and walls with my whiskey bottle between my legs."

"Marine, listen to me." There was silence.

"Where is your weapon?" I requested an answer.

Jimmy replied, "My pistol is on the couch right next to me, friend…fully loaded." He paused. "But all I need is one bullet…haw." He spun what sounded like the cylinder near the handset.

I felt helpless. I knew the more he drank, the drunker he would get and the greater the possibility of suicide. He needed a reason to live. He was calling for help. Sometimes, it just takes someone showing he or she cares whether a person lives or dies. When veterans begin drinking heavily, they become abusive, mostly to themselves, and at times, lash out at others. There is no question suicide becomes a real alternative to them especially if they become sick and tired of being sick and tired. Over a longer period of time drinking and building up a tolerance and needing more alcohol or drugs to reach the same effect, the vet may become dependent on the substance. This becomes a serious heath disorder and requires immediate professional help.

"Jimmy, would you do me a favor, buddy," I asked. "Take the bullets out of the chamber and cylinder of your weapon while you have me on the phone and put them somewhere in your place away from you so we can talk this over? I can't carry on a conversation with you knowing you have a pistol cylinder loaded with bullets, spinning it in my ear. Agreed?"

Jimmy was slow to answer. I could tell he was thinking my question over. I have been here before. The important task at this point is to disarm the warrior and talk him down from harming himself.

I was waiting for his response, I asked again, "Jimmy, will you unload your weapon for me?"

I then asked with urgency and insistence as I needed to disarm him. "Jimmy, talk to me. Do you hear what I am asking you?"

"Yeah," he muttered. "Okay, I will drop the bullets into my hand and put them in my drawer in the kitchen. Is that good enough for you? "

"Yes, buddy, that is good enough. Let me hear the loose bullets in your hand, okay?"

"Wow, you sure are picky, picky. Don't you trust me?" he blurted out.

"I am listening. I want to make sure you are safe, Jimmy. I really do care that you get the help you need—today?" I asked.

He said nothing. Then, I heard him rustling around and some background noise. It sounded like there were bullets in his hand. He left the phone for a minute. I waited. Then, I heard movement near the phone.

"Hello, you still there?" Jimmy belted out.

"Yes, Jimmy, I will not leave you, buddy. I want you to get some help today, right now. Will you come to my clinic and see me today? Can you get a ride in to see me? Do you hear me, Jimmy? I have your back, Marine."

"Well, that's good, Vic, because nobody else has it. All my buddies are dead or out of the service; they disappeared like I did. Yeah! And my wife is gone with another dude. My best friend and battle buddy blew his brains out. I can't sleep without drinking myself into passing out; the nightmares and flashbacks are too much, What a life! Haw! I am going to hang up now, Vic., No more talk," he said hopelessly.

"Wait a minute Jimmy," I jumped in. "Let me give you our medical clinic address. You already have my phone number.' Jimmy agreed, and I gave him the street address information and directions.

"I am leading a veteran's group beginning this week at 6 o'clock pm every Tuesday and Thursday. We have room for two more combat veterans, Jimmy. Will you be there buddy? This group will have vets in need of help just like you. It will be filled with 12 American heroes just like you, Marine. And me. Yes, Jimmy, I am a former Marine Corps rifleman, Vietnam. Hope to see you there."

I heard a click on the line. No words. The phone went dead silent.

I began to think about our conversation, about how Jimmy began to like the smell of death and burned powder. *Did Jimmy really want to die?*

Jill Carroll's article (July 2008), "When the War Comes Back Home," in the *Christian Science Iraq*

*Monitor* immediately came to mind while talking with Jimmy. Once upstanding service members were getting arrested for domestic violence and bar fights and being pursued by police as they raced along streets at 100 miles per hour, often with drugs or alcohol involved, seeking to replicate the adrenaline rush of combat or to commit suicide by motorcycle or police bullets (WJACTV, 2006).

# CHAPTER TEN

# Living Homeless

"I sold my soul to the highest bidder," Corporal Garcia mumbled. Marine Corporal Ruben Garcia, using the stimulating action of methamphetamine to support an inflated sense of self-worth, sat clenching his teeth and wringing his hands while "mad dogging" the other veterans in group room # 2.

It was his turn to speak. The former Marine was out of detox, still suffering from the withdrawal effects of methamphetamine dependence. He looked abnormally thin: sunken cheeks, shiny with sweat.

The 34-year-old Ruben strained to raise a nervous smile as he began to tell his story. "I'm a former Marine "grunt." Fought over in Iraq, Gulf War in 2003. We kicked the Republican Guard's ass. I was on the front lines with the 1st Marine Division when shit hit the fan. Now, sometimes I can't go anywhere without feeling like the enemy is chasing me. I use whatever drugs I can get my hands on to survive the flashbacks, mostly crystal meth."

During my years in graduate school, one college professor assigned Denis Waitley's best-selling book, *Seeds of Greatness* (1988), was required reading. I am forever grateful. Waitley tells the story, "It's Still Me Inside," about a man named Larry who endured more than 60 operations. Dr. Waitley said that even after a year, it was very difficult to look his friend square in the face. Larry had been burned much more severely than Waitley had anticipated. "But to hear him talk about it you would have thought he burned his fingers barbecuing in the backyard!" Waitley went to the physical therapist with his friend and watched him go through the excruciating pain of having his fingers pulled, bent, and massaged so he could move them properly and get the tendons stretched back in the right direction. Waitley wrote in his book, "When he saw me hesitate to talk...eye to eye," Larry said, "Don't worry, buddy. It's still me inside, just a temporary reconstruction job going on at the surface." The author goes on to say, "He told me that if you had faith and really knew yourself from 'inside-out,' you wouldn't get discouraged when something unexpected came along to threaten you from the 'outside-in.'"

"Here was a young man," Dr. Waitley wrote, "with everything going on for him, when suddenly everything went up in smoke. Why was he not crushed or broken? I thought about the thousands of young people who take their lives every year because they are depressed about their inability to cope with change. I thought about the thousands of complaints I have heard in my life from people who just are plain miserable."

Flying back to San Diego, Waitley stared out the airplane window and tried to comprehend his friend's unbelievable attitude. He figured that if you're born in despair, it would be tough to maintain your faith. But Larry's belief was that since he had been born healthy, in America, with a strong spiritual faith, he wasn't going to let an accident discourage him. "It's much easier to get back to being who you know you are than it is to become like someone you don't know.'

So it was with Army Corporal Garcia. He knew who he was before serving in the military. He shared with me over the telephone before coming into the clinic how he was a faithful church youth group leader and believer in the word of God. In fact, he told me that he had read the Holy Bible cover to cover in his teenage years. Ruben yearned for a spiritual transformation; his story shows how to discover your spiritual condition and what to do if you are spiritually bankrupt with no will to live another day. Like many other veterans, the events in Garcia's story can only be described by three words: God's amazing grace.

Ruben is an Army veteran of the Iraq War. He had been homeless since returning to the States from Iraq and was living under a bridge with about 15 other homeless Iraq and Afghanistan veterans. The Corporal had been told he had a "mild" traumatic brain injury (TBI) because of an improvised explosive device (IED) explosion, which the medical doctor said represents a very significant traumatic event. He was unconscious when they got to him.

I learned during my initial face time with Ruben that many other things happened when he experienced his concussion, such as his close buddy was seriously injured, others were killed, and the TBI concussion occurred while in an ambush with the enemy. His medical assessment coming back from deployment indicated that such a close call on his life had led to PTSD. Obviously, he was depressed and feeling hopeless and helpless when he came into see me.

Ruben was giving up. "I lost touch with Jesus," he said somewhat apologetically. "I knew better but I was angry at him. War is a bloody place. I witnessed some tragic stuff, stuff that I can't even begin to forget or express what it did to me. Oh, yes, I had a concussion, but that was not as critical to me as seeing my buddies blow up., Vic. I just can't talk about it; it was horrible. I have tried to put it out of my mind. The medical docs, when they checked me over for my concussion, wanted me to see a shrink, too, but I told them hell no, I'm not weak and helpless. I can handle it." Ruben began to sniffle. I got up from the chair, handed him a Kleenex, went over to my small frig against the wall, and pulled out a small bottle of spring water and handed it to him. I gave him time and returned to my chair. The room fell silent.

Corporal Garcia blew his nose and wiped his face. His feet were flat on the floor; he was sitting straight back in the chair. Ruben sat as if he was at attention. I put my hand on his shoulder. Patting it in a comforting gesture as a comrade in friendship.

I began speaking as his stare directly followed my eyes. "Ruben, you are a good man with a kind heart. I can tell that just in the brief time we have talked together. You are a courageous man, too, and a good and faithful warrior. Welcome home, soldier. Thank you for serving our great nation. I want to help you! I want to begin giving you the help you need right now, right here where you are sitting. Is there any reason why you don't want me to do that?"

I studied his facial features. He had a chiseled jawbone that has seen some rough and tumble action over the years to be sure, large flat nose as in a boxer's, and a thin black mustache groomed down the side of his mouth to a point. He wore polished rawhide boots and jeans with a sizable silver-and-brass buckle. He appeared to keep himself trim and in shape despite the emotional struggles he has been going through.

There was a pause. He was looking down at the floor at his boots.

"Ruben, talk to me, buddy; you have the courage of a warrior. Let me help you!"

"Okay, I am ready. What do I have to do, Vic?" Garcia uttered as he raised both hands to his face, rubbing his perspiration-speckled forehead with the palms of his hands in a circular motion. He twisted and leaned forward slightly toward me.

"You will be just fine," I tried to reassure him. "Hey, this is your chance to get back into the Word. You, my friend, can begin to work on getting the help you need to deal with those haunting memories that have overwhelmed your very soul, right?"

"That sounds good to me, Vic. It is my new mission," he said apprehensively.

"Ok, Ruben, your first step in your recovery action plan is to be sure you get back here, down the hall, at 6 o'clock in group room #2 for a 90-minute vet group. There are 11 other combat veterans in the group. You will fit right in."

I added, "Ruben, I wish you the best life has to offer, buddy. Oorah! Good work today. Oh, by the way, make sure you read John 3:16 again. This is a new start for you."

As I stood and then moved toward the door, I said, "Goodbye, for now. See you tonight. I will be leading the group." I extended my hand and opened the door.

Ruben left the room, heading down the hall when I stuck my head out the door, shouting out and pointing toward group room #2, "Room 2 is right over there, buddy. See you tonight. He smiled, looking back toward me, waving.

A few weeks into Rubens recovery plan I opened the group conversation saying, "How is the world treating you, Ruben?" He looked me square in the eyes smiling.

"I want to thank you for what you did for me, Vic. You gave me hope. You encouraged me. And God did the rest. You wouldn't believe what I am doing now." I could tell Ruben was building up steam in this conversation. I couldn't believe my ears. *This is a new man*, I thought.

It turned out that Ruben went back to church and renewed his commitment to God. He began praying for a renewed spirit to serve. He started gathering donated Bibles from churches in the community and passed them out to his buddies under the bridge that not so many months prior he had called home. He began a Bible study under the bridge, and other homeless veterans and non-vets started to gather, reading and studying the Word of God. Ruben told me he taught mostly from the Book of John found in the New Testament. "It is a book that explains in great detail about the truth and life of Jesus Christ. I found an unconditional love that healed my mind and body and transformed me." Later, I thought about the amazing transformation Ruben had experienced. He had lost all hope of living. He was haunted day and night by the heartfelt scars of losing his buddies in battle. At times, he felt guilty for surviving the bomb blast.

The fact that he chose to seek professional help and get out of his depressed stupor was absolutely uplifting. *This is what I come to work hoping to accomplish every day*, I mused thoughtfully. This is what makes me eager to get started when my feet hit the floor each morning. But I know deep inside the transformation I witnessed was not me making the difference in Chuck's life but rather his faith in a power greater than himself. Ruben is a Christian believer, a combat veteran who lost his way and now has found it once again.

Rick Warren, author of *The Purpose-Driven Life* (2002) and founding pastor of one of the largest and most well-known churches in California, writes: "You are not an accident. Even before the universe was created, God had you in mind, and he planned you for his purposes. These purposes will extend far beyond the few years you will spend on earth. You were made to last forever!

So it was for Ruben. He found his purpose. He was led to spread the Word and inspiration of God to the lost and forsaken few; in his case, these were the homeless veterans and others living under the bridge in his town.

Inspirational Encouragement

Religious counselors frequently carry the burden of grief resolution. Many priests, ministers and rabbis are experienced and comfortable in the role of bereavement counselor. When acceptable and solicited, the implications of the existence of an all-forgiving, all-knowing, loving God who is the ultimate spiritual resource may offer security and hope as well as strength to tolerate the painful effects that afflict the veteran survivors of traumatic combat experiences.

In a magnificent book I read when I was younger, *The Greatest Salesman in the World* (1985), Og Mandino writes:

> Can sand flow upward in the hourglass? Will the sunrise
> where it sets and set where it rises? Can I relive the errors
> of yesterday and right them? Can I call back yesterday's

wounds and make them whole? Can I become younger than yesterday? Can I take back the evil that was spoken, the blows that were struck, and the pain that was caused? No. Yesterday is buried for-ever and I will think of it no more. I will live this day as if it is my last (p. 105).

A favorite of mine! Spencer Johnson, M.D., is one of the country's most sought-after thinkers and admired authors. Dr. Johnson earned a B.A. degree in Psychology from the University of Southern California, an M.D. degree from the Royal College of Surgeons, and medical clerkships at The Mayo Clinic and Harvard Medical School. More than forty-six million copies of Spencer Johnson's books are in print worldwide in more than forty-seven languages.

I have had enormous success teaching and counseling on the true value of living in the present. Focusing on the here and now in treatment and action plans more for today, navigating veterans away from living in the past and focusing more on the present. Who you are right now because who you are is precious, And you are the present.

I hope these two messages inspire you as they have me.

# CHAPTER 11

# A Sniper Haunted

I saw Marine Sergeant Joe Mendez Joe sitting in the waiting room for an appointment I set up after I had talked with him at length earlier in the day. A sight for sore eyes, to use a cliché, he wore faded camo pants and military boots worn from back in the day in country. As I approached, I saw a square, powerful-looking man with piercingly black eyes and faded-rust hair. His worn, original-issue camo hat tilted forward on his head.

Joe looked at me coming toward him across the waiting room and partially smiled, a tooth missing and others crooked and worn. We introduced ourselves and shook hands. I felt my knuckles pop and grind. Hello!

Later that same evening, 59-year-old former Marine Sergeant, 3rd Marine Division, and scout sniper Joe Mendez angrily told the other seasoned warriors in group room #2, "Speed-balling is the curse God put on my life. " Joe was so filled with pent-up emotions from killing experiences in 1970 Vietnam still haunting him more than four decades after returning home to a divided America that he literally spit with rage when he spoke.

If a warrior allows emotions to seep in, he or she runs the risk of becoming a liability to the others on the mission. In the heat of battle, adrenaline kicks in as well. This "blood lust" can damage a warrior's soul for a lifetime. The guilty feelings associated with killing other human beings can be enormous and haunt the veteran warrior for many years after the combat experience. Many veterans express feelings of guilt because they enjoyed the hunt and the kill.

Earlier in the day, for a brief moment, I had walked out of my office down the hall and looked out of the huge, red brick-lined window just to the left of my door. Suddenly, not two minutes into my walk, my phone rang. Immediately, I scurried quickly back to pick up the call at my desk.

A gruff voice came on the line. "I feel like killing myself right here, right now!" The voice on the other end of the line said, wheezing heavily.

"Hello, my name is Vic. What is your name?" I asked kindly.

"Joe, the man, pretty sick in the head, I think. I've tried to hold on for all these years, Vic. I have outlasted the NVA's artillery shelling, land mines, booby traps, snipers, mortar attacks, ambushes. Got out of there carrying my balls on a stretcher. Lived in the mountains of Colorado, Idaho and Wyoming. For the life of me, can't remember how many years; moved around most of the United States, Canada, and Mexico at times. Shit!" The caller paused, out of breath.

"I am tired. Just tired of living. I guess what I'm saying. it finally has whipped me. It's over, man. I'm dead meat. Never had a home to call mine, Vic. Never had a family to welcome me back home; still have no family, no kids, no wife. Oh, I had bed partners here and there, but no permanent 'ol' lady', you understand. I can't get close to nobody. I've never been right since Nam. I know it. Hell, I don't need a doctor to tell me shit!" Joe sounded anxious as he unloaded a pound of pent-up emotion until he literally ran out of breath. He was swallowing heavily, gulping, and obviously having a difficult time breathing.

I interrupted, with some worry, and finally got a word in, "Wow, buddy, it sounds to me like you just about covered it. Let me ask you, have you hurt yourself tonight?"

"No," he paused. "Not yet, but I have a razor blade to do the job. Just fill up some hot water and let her bleed. I have thought about that. Not afraid to cut myself. Shit, in Khe Sanh we did everything, saw everything, and felt nothin'. I saw guts lying out on the ground of some new recruit who stepped on a 'mouse trap' AP mine. He was still alive, looking around, crying out for his mommy. It don't mean nothin'.' I didn't even know his name. He joined our team a couple of days before, real green. He looked something like my kid brother. He looked at me as if I could do something for him. Hell, he was lying there in his own blood and guts, waiting to die. I couldn't do nothin'. He was trying to put himself back together, stuffing his own intestines back into the wound hole in his belly. I wanted to help him stuff it back in, but I knew it was only a matter of minutes, too late for a medevac. I called for a corpsman, anyway. Told the kid he would be alright; the medic was on his way. That's all I could do. We lie to our dying comrades every time, letting them think there is hope for them, but we know it is over, man. I still see his hazy face in my dreams. I have had to live with this shit since 1968...forty f—in' years, man...just too much to live with," Joe agonized.

I responded quickly. I wanted to let him know someone out there cared. "Welcome home, Joe. Long time overdue, buddy, but welcome home," I said, somewhat apologizing for our country's lack of response to our returning heroes.

"Thank you for serving our country," I added.

Joe did not respond. No words were spoken by either of us for a moment. I felt a burst of sadness right then. Tears welled up in my eyes as I looked down at my yellow notepad on the desk, a couple of water spots soaking into the paper, waiting for the right time to speak again. I felt for this broken, suffering vet. The lonely years of torment—he must have been in absolute misery.

*If only he will come into the clinic for counseling,* I mused. *What a tragedy! Time is of the* essence.

Former president of the United States Herbert Hoover once was quoted as saying: "Older men declare war. But it is youth that must fight and die. And it is youth who must inherit the tribulation, the sorrow, and the triumphs that are the aftermath of war."

Then, I heard a congested voice on the other end of the line. "Yeah, thanks Vic," Joe voiced quietly.

"Joe, we can help you now. It isn't too late for you, buddy. There is a lot of support for Nam, Iraq and Afghanistan combat vets today. Your call to me is just a starting point for you. I can get you connected to a VA nearest to you, right now. There are trained counselors and therapists who can work with you and help you find solutions to overcome your feelings of hopelessness and wanting to end your life prematurely," I pleaded earnestly. "Will you let me get you help?"

"Too late, Vic," Joe said apologetically.

"What do mean, 'too late'?" my voice rose. "Talk to me, Joe!"

"I mean I have already made up my mind," he responded determinedly.

"Why, then, did you call me today?" I asked in order to reach out to him.

"I just needed to tell someone. I am all alone and wanted someone to know I was checking out," he said sadly.

"Tell me what specifically, Joe. What do you want to tell me? I am listening, buddy; talk to me. Where is the pain?" I asked directly.

He replied softly, "I was drafted. I had no choice but to go. I have always been against brutality and feel so guilty about the killing I had to do in the war. I had to survive. I had to fight back or die. I was there; my squad was counting on me. Do you understand, Vic? I had to defend myself. I had to complete the mission." Joe spoke as if he were looking for forgiveness.

"I mean, it seems like I am numb inside all the time. I have these dreams and thoughts about some of the KIA bodies I saw: the gurgling noises from their mouths and look of their faces—at the end, all distorted. I can't forget those death stares. The scenes I saw, the destruction I witnessed. I don't think there has been a day gone by, in all these years, that I don't think about that kid with his gut pouring out and the nightmares...even sweats. I am tired, Vic, bone tired."

"Joe, can I ask you to do something for me?" I said with feeling.

"What's that?" he quickly replied.

"Would you please put the razor blade away, somewhere safe and out of reach while we continue to talk about things? Is there any reason you can't do that for me, buddy?" I requested intently. No immediate response from the tired warrior. I waited, looking up at the wall clock, thinking about what I knew about assessing suicide risk factors, including

- Does the veteran have the desire to kill himself? Joe had the desire to kill himself. He already expressed those feelings.
- What kind of feelings does the veteran express? Is the veteran depressed and hopeless? Joe stated he felt hopeless and intolerably alone. He described the psychological pain, the intense misery he had to live with for so many years.
- Does the veteran seem likely to and capable of hurting himself? Joe had the capability and sense of fearlessness to try. He said, "I'm not afraid to cut me." He was also demonstrating increased anxiety.

- Does the veteran have a specific plan and the opportunity for an attempt? Yes, Joe had both a plan and the opportunity for a suicide attempt.

- Has the veteran thought out the details? Joe had acquired the means (a razor blade) to follow through on his plan.

- Has the veteran prepared for the finality of death? Has the veteran written any notes or given away possessions? (This is a very important sign for suicide intent.)Unknown at the time for Joe's case.

- Does the veteran have a support system (family, friends) to connect to or is he alone? Joe had explained he had no family, children, or wife; that he "can't get close to nobody."

- Does the veteran talk about plans or does he have no plans? Joe had expressed, "I have no reason for living."

- Does the veteran convey a sense of purpose? Joe was expressing no sense of purpose.

- Is the veteran undecided about dying? Joe was not undecided about dying; he knew he wanted it (Baldwin, 2007).

Based on these factors, if one decided to pick up the phone and dial 911 based on the Risk Factors for Joe, that would be the correct decision.

Joe began to talk. "Why should I put the blade away since I am going to use it?" he asked somberly.

"Wait one minute, Joe! You do have reasons to live, and I will tell you why," I exclaimed.

Joe snapped back, "you tell me what this over-the-hill has-been has to offer anyone. I am worthless, Vic. Haven't you been listening to a word I have been saying? Shit, man, you don't get it, do you?" Joe recoiled.

"I get it, Joe. Now, will you give me a minute and I will tell you why I think you have a reason to live. What do you mean when you said you can't get close to anybody?" I prompted him to respond.

"Nobody knows how I bleed inside every time I think or dream about the combat deaths and mutilation. All the carnage I saw and was part of in Vietnam still controls my thoughts, Vic." Joe paused for a moment. I heard some commotion in the background. Then, I heard a whishing sound near the receiver. It sounded like he took a drag between his lips from a cigarette. *Hmm, I wonder if he is self-medicating with cannabis weed. Is he addicted? Does he take any other meds?*

Joe started talking again before I could jump in.

"I feel unsafe all the time. I walk outside, and loud noises from the street upset me. I never know what to expect. When I was in-country, the gook's artillery barrage was pounding, but at least I knew it was going to rain rockets—and I always had a hole in the ground or hooch to jump into. But now I worry about protecting myself, watchin' my own back from people, noises, and bad situations. So, I don't go out much. I try to stay to what is familiar to me. I feel safer that way, Vic."

*Joe showed signs of slowing down in his conversation. It probably is the effect of the pot,* I mused. *What is my next plan of action?* I thought, *I must talk him down from a suicide attempt. How am I going to accomplish that? I must stay focused and continue talking to him about the reasons he must live.*

"Joe, do you ever get to the VA in your area?" I asked.

"Hell no, I had enough of the freakin' VA back in the '60s and '70s. They gave me nothin' but more pain. Couldn't trust them. 'Take three aspirins and see me in a couple months.' And did I have nightmares big time. Some of the veteran old-timers called it 'shell shock' from all the mortars and rockets pounding us into the ground. That was tough sleddin' back then. I headed for the mountains with a couple of buddies when we got out but could never get away from the noises in my head," Joe expounded.

"Joe, let's talk, buddy, about putting that razor blade away and letting me get you some help. I will arrange for you to talk with good people at the VA. You will be able to talk to other combat vets also from Vietnam and the wars in Iraq and Afghanistan—many going through the same or similar as you. The treatment teams today are highly trained at treating combat trauma, not just medical doctors. The VA team will develop a treatment plan for you that will help you make sense of and understand your emotions and help you to get in touch with those feelings of guilt and fear," I said, arguing for his life. "We are talking about freedom, Joe. Freedom for you to be able to get out of the house and go places, meet people, make new friends, and maybe find a special lady. These are just a few of the reasons why I want you to help me help you."

Joe responded, "Nope. Thanks, but no thanks. I can handle this.

"I care about what happens to you, buddy. Semper Fi. I have your back if you will let me," I pleaded, hoping he would respond in kind.

"You a leatherneck, Vic? No shit! What the hell, you are, aren't you? Semper Fi back at you, bro," he replied with a level of surprise and exuberance in his voice.

"Joe, I will give you another reason to live: your Marine buddies who died in Khe Sanh. Wouldn't they want you to live…for them, Joe…in their memory? Wouldn't they want you to help other vets from other wars recover, giving them strength and hope to overcome from their wounds?" I asked.

I had to be careful here not to transfer a burden of guilt on to Joe's shoulders. I wanted to give him a sense of purpose, encourage a mission.

"Joe, you would have an enormous effect on these young warriors coming home from Iraq and Afghanistan. Once you work through your issues and begin to get your mental and physical health back, sharing and caring is what recovery is all about. This is for you, buddy. I know you don't think you want this right now, but I am truly hoping you will get the help you need and deserve. I know you said you don't like the VA so how about coming in to my clinic and meet with me today. Oorah!"

"You will see me now, Vic?" Joe said with a sense of hopefulness in his voice.

"Yes, Marine, I can see you later today. Let's get'er done! We have room in a veteran's group at 6 o'clock Tuesdays and Thursdays. Tonight, how about coming to see me before group, say at 4:30, We can talk privately and get some good face-to-face time, getting to know each other, Joe. I would like that, buddy. When we are done, then I lead the combat vets group at 6:00. What do you think?

"I will be there, Vic! I'm so sick and tired of being sick and tired, bro. Thanks for caring, man. See you at 4:30." Joe hung up the phone.

A generalized therapeutic model for recovery from combat trauma suggests that before Joe can begin to heal from remembering and dreaming about his feelings associated with experiences on the battlefield, he must first become more comfortable with his internal and external safety zones. Joe must come to terms and learn to process feelings associated with his exterior environment as well as within his wounded soul. Once he finds safety in his environment and in his consciousness, he can begin to repair and rebuild the sensitive feelings and behaviors associated with his guilt. These hinge on the feelings of remorse and depression he discussed as well as the grief and anger that come with them.

# CHAPTER 12

# A Military Secret

It is a well-kept secret that a significant percentage of combat troops, in the war zones, are medicated with psychiatric drugs to facilitate their continuing to carry out stressful, deadly, and sometimes daily missions. In fact, psychiatric drugs are being prescribed, consumed, shared, and traded in combat zones. Many warriors then return stateside, chemically dependent on those antipsychotic, anti-anxiety drugs and sleeping pills. Forty-two-year-old Marine Sergeant Russell Mason of the 1st Armored Division, Machine Gunner, Desert Storm, Gulf War was no exception. He, too, had trouble getting to sleep and calming his post-traumatic stress and was prescribed psychiatric drugs. Russ was referred to the clinic by the VA Medical Center and needed help learning to relax enough to be able to readjust to civilian life back home–without drugs.

Sometimes, the immediate intervention and treatment of a veteran is critical. Veterans need guidance to learn how to connect with other veterans coping with the same or similar challenges. Another veteran can provide the encouragement and support an emotionally challenged veteran needs to begin the process of overcoming obstacles and healing. (A list of VA Resources for this purpose is provided in Appendix B.)

As soon as I heard his voice, I knew he was troubled and quickly responded, "Russ, I am glad you called the clinic today, buddy. Thanks for serving our country. Welcome home. How may I help you?" I asked.

"Welcome home, my ass! I have no home! No reason to live," Russ agonized loudly, spitting the words into the telephone receiver. "I have no money and no gas to get out of this stinking trailer park parking lot; no one will hire me; I have no food; I am living in my truck. I am tired of all this f—n' shit. I served my time for this country! No one cares about what happens to me."

Russ was 100% disabled and needed someone to talk to, someone to reach out to or, more important, he needed someone to reach out to him. Russ apparently was not aware of his vulnerability of being seduced by suicide ideation. He had isolated himself from his family and friends and seldom went out into the community. He was on prescription medication for bipolar disorder. Sam suffered from a combat and alcohol-induced mood disorder in addition to mood swings from mania. This showed up as exaggerated feelings of well-being or stimulation. In such moods, a vet can lose touch with reality and, following the mania, feel acute depression, which Russ described as "engulfing me with overwhelming feelings of sadness and anxiety."

"Are you thinking about suicide, Russ?" I questioned. "Maybe just need help? Someone to talk to?"

"I'm sitting here in my truck, and I'm tired of living like this," he said, sounding a bit more approachable.

"What led you to call this number?" I asked. *I need to know the reason Russ dialed this number today*, I thought, waiting for his response.

"I get pretty sad, down in the dumps most days." He paused. I could hear him drinking something, then puffing on something, inhaling and exhaling. *Most likely a cigarette or weed*, I thought.

He continued after a loud swallow, "I feel shitty most of the time. I'm mentally challenged. That's no big deal, but I feel trapped sometimes. That sucks. Nothing to do, nowhere to go, no one to visit or talk to. What kind of life is this?" Russ stopped talking abruptly. I heard nothing and then another sound in the background—a shuffling or something moving. I could hear what sounded like the truck door closing.

"Hello, Russ? Hey, buddy, are you there?" Nothing but silence.

"Talk to me, Russ. Hello?" *What is happening?* I thought. *Why did he leave so quickly? Did he get out of his truck?* He said nothing. *The phoneline is still open; where did he go?* I thought. I waited. I sat with my elbows on the desk, head held in my hands, eyes looking straight down at my yellow notepad. I drew a large question mark with my pencil.

I looked up, glancing in the direction of the clock—I looked back down at my notepad. I doodled around my notes. I had written a few scribbles as I was talking to Russ. I jotted down another note: "Mixing alcohol with prescription drugs…big problem!!" I wrote with big, double exclamation marks and circled. This could be more serious than Russ realizes, even a possible overdose, a non-intentional suicide. Mixing drugs for depression and anxiety with the depressive effects of alcohol is not a good thing. *Where is he? He probably would have hung up the phone if the call was over, but would he think to hang up the phone in his present state of mind, depressed and possibly suicidal? What's going on?*

My experience and training as a crisis line interventionist has taught me that the common psychological denominator in nearly all suicides is depression, the miserable mood that causes the colors of life to fade. Chronically depressed individuals who have never known a day of happiness live with an inconsolable disappointment and sadness that makes existence meaningless and hopeless. Despondent veterans are convinced that they are at the mercy of unfavorable circumstances affecting their existences. On a more severe level, manic-depressive veterans categorized as bipolar are a population highly vulnerable to self-destruction in the depressed phase. Russell appeared to be alienated from others, unable to socialize and psychological barriers prevented him from accessing support from people in the community. Alcoholism—as often as all other maladaptive instances put together—is the agent most likely to lead to suicide. Russ sounded as though he was intoxicated or at the very least high on some mind-altering substance.

I continued holding my phone receiver listening to the open telephone line. *Where did Russ go? Why did he not say something to me if he was leaving?*

Suddenly, I heard the truck door open; I sensed some sort of motion. I waited to hear a voice, Russ's voice, but all that filled the line emptiness. I couldn't imagine what was happening. *Why isn't Russ talking to me? Decision time! Do I send the police? Better safe than sorry,* I thought. *But I have no sound criteria that Russ is in trouble; depressed probably, but suicidal? Not sure. And I don't have a clue where he is calling from. I need more information.*

Then, I heard some more commotion, and Russ broke the silence, "Hello! Are you still there?"

"I am here, Russ…still here, buddy. What is happening? Have you done anything to hurt yourself?"

"Nope. Just took a leak behind a big old' tree." he began. "Hurt myself? Well, let me see, I am buzzed on pot, drunk on booze, and medicated on different colored pills for my so-called bipolar thing. What the hell! Does that sound like I am hurting myself, dude?"

"Have you ever attempted suicide, Russ?" I asked.

No immediate answer, then Russ responded, "Not really. Well, I think I know what is going to happen to me if I keep going on like this, I mean drinking so much…the pills, the weed. Some days, I really don't want to wake up, you know. Just getting tired of being depressed.

"Tell me more about your 'not wanting to get up in the morning' thoughts, Russ. What has been happening in your life recently to make you want to give up?" I probed for more information.

"I told you: I have no money, just a few bucks from my lousy disability check. I am stuck here! Right here, right now." Russ was getting agitated. I decided to back off. He continued, "Every day since I got back home from the war games in the desert, haw," he retorted, "I've been homeless or living in low-life motels and in the cheap, cheap boarding houserooms until the money runs out. Then, I sleep in my truck until the next check comes to my post office general delivery. It all started 18 years ago, dude. Now, same ol', same ol'. Nothing changes; same s—, different day." He paused for a breath.

"Have you tried to get more help for your situation?" I asked.

"Help from where? Hell, I was in the Battle of Medina Ridge in Desert Storm with the kick-ass 1st Armored Division that kicked Iraqi Republican Guard's proverbial butt. Yeah, hmm," he paused, and it sounded like he took another drink, gulping it down. "I was a part of the largest tank battle in U.S. history, dude. I was part of it. A big deal to tell my grandkids, huh? Yeah, kiddies, your grandpa was a gunner on a Bradley fighting machine in Iraq. I fought close range—lots of noise and machine guns. I watched some real blood and guts, Iraqis on fire, running, yelling. So, I shot them." He paused and cleared his throat. "That's what I do as a gunner. I shoot cannons and machine guns. I am a real tough guy."

Russ stopped talking, I could hear him take another swig from his bottle. I had nothing to say at this point. I was transfixed on what he had just said about his grandchildren. All I could do was listen as he continued to ramble.

"Only problem is this tough guy has no family, no grandkids. When I returned home, I was 24 years old. My girlfriend who said she would wait for me married someone else; wonderful surprise," Russ said sarcastically. "Oh, did I mention my family kicked me out of the house after a few months because I was 'behaving strangely'? Imagine that—my own flesh and blood booted me out, the ultimate dagger through the heart. So, here we are, dude, just you and me, and I don't even know your name."

"Vic is my name, Russ. Vic Montgomery, former Marine, the Nam, buddy. Oorah!" I have your back. How can I help you?"

"Jarhead, huh? Devil Dog? Oorah, Vic!" he responded as if a barrier had been lifted.

"We really need to talk about how I can get you the help you need, Russ," I replied.

"Well," he slurred, the effects of the drugs and alcohol becoming more apparent, "to answer your earlier question, yes, I have already been to the VA psych docs and others several years back. I took some tests; they gave me some suicide screenings and scripts. That was about it, end of story. I'm still here. I used to go in about every three months for refills and a five-minute chat with the doc, but I don't see the need for that anymore," he said antagonistically. "I have no love for some of these docs and nurses from foreign countries. Half the time I don't understand what they are saying. I am sure they are okay guys and gals, but what the hell happened to our American doctors and nurses?" he expounded.

"What about you right now, Russ? Do you have any specific plan to hurt yourself?" I asked deliberately.

"I'm doing it, brother! Right in front of you," he insisted.

"What are you doing, Russ?"

"Hell, I hurt myself every day, Vic. Who the hell cares?" he said harshly.

"You're drinking?" I said, questioning his metaphorical statement.

"I've lost my will to live, Vic. I am giving up, partner. No more, man." Russ was beginning to bow out of this conversation.

"Russ, where are you located right now? Where is the trailer park? "I insisted.

"What do you mean trailer park? How do you know that?" he questioned, somewhat paranoid.

"Earlier you said you were parked on a lot in a trailer park, living in your truck," I replied.

"Oh, yeah, I forgot I told you that. It is called the Shady Oak Trailer Park. Why do you want to know?" he asked.

"Because I want to send you some help to get you to the VA hospital," I responded.

"Send me help! What, are you crazy? First of all, this place is so small it doesn't have an address, and no one will ever be able to find me out here. Yo! That's why I'm here. And another thing, how do you know what I need? You are on a telephone, God knows where." Russ challenged.

"Maybe I don't know exactly what you need, Russ, so I am hoping you can help me help you," I suggested. "How about it, Russ? You help me understand— things like how much drinking and drugging you do. How much and how often, Russ?" I asked sincerely.

"Who's counting?" he replied quickly.

"Russ, you called me, right? In a way you are asking for help, right?" I questioned.

"Maybe …," he remarked quietly. I heard him take another drink from his bottle.

"So, you are drinking yourself to death. Is that an accurate statement?" I asked.

"Probably," he said.

"So, Russ, do you think you are suffering from alcoholism?" I asked.

"I guess so, now that you put it that way," he said rather reluctantly.

"Have you thought about why you are drinking yourself to death? "I asked.

There was no immediate response, then he offered half-heartedly, "I have a lot of guilt about the killing I did in Iraq. At times, I can't control my feelings. I cry out of the blue. Sometimes, I can't control it or shut it off. How embarrassing is that? This tough guy, war veteran, a crybaby? I don't enjoy things anymore. I can't sleep. I feel empty most of the time."

WebMD (2009) states: "The severity of the depressive and manic phases of bipolar disorder can differ from person to person and in the same person at different times." In fact, as WebMD suggests, manic phases can lead to drug and alcohol abuse and, as well, depressive phases can present as crying uncontrollably, expressing feelings of hopelessness and worthlessness and thoughts of death and suicide.

As I listened to Russ pour out his feelings of quiet desperation, I realized he was getting drunker and drunker as we talked and more depressed as time slipped past. I had to initiate a plan of action to get him to safety. The only way to find Russ and negotiate an emergency rescue would be for him to tell me the name of the closest city or town. When Russ paused, I interjected calmly, "I care about you, buddy. Really do. You deserve to have a good life ahead of you. And to play with grandchildren. You served our country with honor and courage, Russ. Those depressive feelings of hopelessness and out-of-control crying you describe are treatable, and there is a way out from under the dark cloud of gloom you just shared with me. I feel your pain, buddy. I have your back if you will let me help you. I know you would do the same for me, wouldn't you, Russ?" I asked purposefully.

"Oorah," came Russ's garbled response.

"Sergeant, listen to me. There are professional treatment teams exactly for your situation that will help you work through these haunting experiences you described. You can get over this wall, Russ." I wanted so much to extend my hand to him, to pull him up through this stressful time. "Hey, Russ, I remember when I went through the Marine Corps boot camp PT course, there was always a high wooden wall or two or three, looked like ten or twelve feet high, and the object was to help your squad, rifle team, climb over the wall with full packs and rifle. Remember those boot camp days, buddy?" I said hoping for some sort of response.

"Oorah ...," he said more faintly now.

"Well, what a feat," I continued, "and of course it was impossible to get over the wall without help from your buddies. Right? So, we offered our backs, knees, and shoulders, hand-in-hand, anything to get over the wall."

*So here I am*, I thought, *wanting to give this warrior a hand to get over his wall of discouragement. He is slipping away; I must act quickly. I don't know if he is only intoxicated or if there are more drugs involved.*

"Russ, listen to me, buddy. I want to help you get over the wall right now. I want to send you an emergency rescue team to pick you up and take you to the closest hospital for an emergency evaluation. I fear you may have hurt yourself, buddy. We can't wait any longer. Do you hear what I am saying? Do you understand me?"

"Okay, dude …," his voice was fainter. *I am losing him.*

"Then, we can arrange for transport to the nearest VA Medical Center, get you connected with the VA's crisis prevention coordinator, and the treatment team will see to it you are referred for proper care for your depression and alcohol abuse. Which VA Medical Center do you go to, Russ? Quickly man."

"A VA Center somewhere…if anyone gives a s—," he spoke loudly into the telephone.

I needed to contact because Russ did not know his location. I had to try to find Shady Oak Trailer Park and get to Russ before it was too late. I worried about an accidental overdose. Russ has been drinking a lot. Many suicides happen accidentally. I know Russ also had prescribed anti-depressant medication and who knows what else.

"Russ, are you still with me, buddy?" I asked.

"Yeah, dude, what's happening?" he slurred.

"Russ, I need some help here. What kind of truck are you in right now?" I pleaded to him for assistance.

"Chevy pickup with a camper shell, if you have to know," he said, sounding a bit put off and garbled, as if he had just taken another swallow of booze from his bottle.

"What color and license plate number, Russ?" I asserted.

"Blue. I don't know my license plate number." Russ said.

"How about getting out of the truck and looking?"

"I can't move." He said incoherently.

I wrote this information on my notepad and circled it with my pencil, underlining blue pickup with camper shell and Shady Oak Trailer Park as well as the cell phone number we had obtained with caller ID. It was important for me to stay on the line with Russ so I had contacted one of our staff admin and handed him a note with the specifics of the Sheriff's Department. Our clinic staff indicated he was on the line with the sheriff trying to find the Shady Oak Trailer Park. However, the sheriff did not know such a trailer park the general vicinity nor had anyone figured out where it was located. So far, no one knew where Russ was parked.

"Russ," I called into my telephone handset. No response.

I spoke again, "Russ!" Silence. I mean a dead silence, no static, nothing.

"Russ, buddy, hang in there with me. I have help on the way. Come on, Russ, you must meet me halfway on this, buddy. Talk to me!" I said with emphasis. I was very worried. *Have I lost contact with this troubled veteran?* I asked myself. *Has his cell phone run out of juice? What is happening with Sam? Is the rescue too little too late? I should have pulled an intervention much sooner; why did I hesitate? Come on law enforcement! I can't believe no one knows the name of this trailer park. Come on, guys, give me something.*

I waited a few minutes then, getting up from my desk, I rushed to the admin office next to mine. Dipped in the doorway, I asked, "Anything?"

He shook his head. "Nothing yet; nobody knows where this place is. One sheriff deputy officer thought it may be in another county north of them. We have asked to be transferred, and we are waiting."

"Keep up the good work, team. Let's find this vet." I tried to motivate them, but I found little strength in my delivery. I was physically and mentally drained at this point.

The staff knows how frustrating these moments in limbo can be for the crisis interventionists and the urgency of the matter. This is life-and-death on the line, and they realize it.

I returned to my desk. I couldn't sit down. I paced around the room, looking up at the foreboding clock on the wall. Because of the nature of what we do, time can work against us. I looked in the direction of the admin office. I was looking for some kind of sign they had contacted someone; any news at this point would be, at least, encouraging. I just wanted to know if the location Russ even mentioned actually existed. *Is this a real place or did Russ steer me in the wrong direction…on purpose? Maybe he didn't want to be rescued? Maybe he just wanted someone to hear his story before he killed himself.*

I waited.

Finally, the call came into the clinic. A sheriff deputy in a rural county knew where the small, obscure trailer park was located and was enroute to that location with an ambulance. I urged staff to communicate to the deputy that this intoxicated veteran might be unconscious and in need of emergency medical attention. I also informed them to pass on to the deputy that this vet was already a patient at a VA Medical Center but not sure which location.

*Time for a break.* I contemplated. I turned and walked down the hall into the break room feeling satisfied we'd taken a huge first step to getting this vet to safety.

While in the break room, I leaned back in a chair against the wall, briefly looking up at the wall-mounted television that was blaring some current events news show. As I stared at the screen, I realized I was not hearing or seeing anything. My mind was too involved in wondering whether the rescuers had reached Russ in time.

After a few minutes, I quickly rose from my chair, threw my coffee into the sink, and headed back to my office. I entered the doorway and approached my desk, glancing in the direction of the admin office. One of the staff, apparently hearing me enter the room, returned my glance but did not give me any indication whether the rescue had been made. I sat down on the end of my desk, my phone line still in a holding pattern. I looked up at the clock on the wall; it had been at least 45 minutes since our last contact with the deputy sheriff. I stood up and walked toward the other office, passing several desks on the way. Everyone knows when someone on the team has a rescue in progress; the action is intense.

The team "on rescue" and in pursuit is always up and moving, handing notes, and checking on data and telecom communications. Heads bob and weave in and out and around communication terminal desktops and office doorways. All designated lines are open to the sheriff's department in the veteran's geographic area. Law enforcement has always been first-rate about keeping the intervention team advised of up-to-the-minute information about the rescue and particularly where they are in relation to the warrior in need. In Russ's case, we received a call from the sheriff unit saying they had just arrived at the trailer park and were beginning to search for the pickup truck. Our team had passed on the information I supplied: Russ's name and the fact he may have passed out while talking to me due to intoxication or that he may have harmed himself in a suicide attempt; either case was a real possibility. It was vital for our team to pass on to the paramedics the information that Russ may have taken other drugs as well as alcohol. It was confirmed that the sheriff was accompanied by an ambulance and paramedics at our request.

We waited. Then the long-awaited call came in. The sheriff deputies were approaching the camper truck from the rear. They told us they had to use extreme caution in approaching the vehicle because they did not know if there were any weapons inside. The deputies reported no movement inside the truck—no sign of anyone sitting up in the cab or in the back camper shell.

The phones went silent. We waited on hold on the direct line to the sheriff. Minutes passed.

We then received word the sheriff had found Russ's body slumped down near the floorboards on the passenger side, so it had been hard to see him in the cab. The doors were unlocked, and the windows open partially, so it was easy to get Russ out quickly and into the ambulance. After some time spent in giving medical assistance to Russ, the paramedics reported he was in critical condition and had to be transported quickly to the nearest hospital. Apparently, from the medical information relayed to us, Russ may have been in an alcohol-induced coma.

Dr. Debra Emmite, MD is a Psychiatry Specialist in Houston, TX and has over 42 years of experience in the medical field. She has specialized in treating combat war veterans with chemical dependency consequences for many of those years. In Debra Emmite's extended time spent with battle buddies has often suggested in rare instances, excessive alcohol consumption can cause potentially fatal complications that require emergency medical treatment. Alcohol poisoning, or acute intoxication, can cause liver and/or respiratory failure, which may result in heart failure. When a person consumes large amounts of alcohol in a short period of time, "the blood alcohol level rises so high and so quickly that the liver cannot metabolize the alcohol. The person may become comatose, may suffer cardiac and respiratory failure, and can die. In such cases, emergency medical support can be lifesaving.

Russ was on his way to a community hospital nearest to the trailer park location. The paramedics did not want to chance a long trip to get him into an emergency room intensive care unit. From there, the VA crisis prevention coordinators arranged transport to the nearest VA Medical Center for further treatment and level of care follow-up. Russ was fortunate. He made it and was detoxified over a 14-day period after coming out of his coma.

For many alcohol- and other-drug-dependent veterans, detoxification is only the first step in treatment. Detoxification is more than just physical readjustment; it also involves psychological readjustments.

These psychological changes are important as the veteran continues treatment. Veterans struggling with problems that developed prior to substance dependency—for example, broken marriages, reintegration to civilian life from the military, combat trauma, or psychiatric disorders—need continued care and services after detoxification to address these other problems. Detoxification without follow-up care can lead to previous mental and physical health issues going untreated and may result in relapses or other complications.

The special services that Russ had available to him included an intensive inpatient alcohol and drug treatment program for his ongoing recovery treatment planning for addictions and chemical dependency, aftercare and transitional housing referrals, Vet Center support groups for combat veterans, and outpatient counseling and group therapy helping him process his war experiences as well as providing guidance to help him find balance and happiness in his personal life.

After a period, Russ requested to be referred and transferred to our outpatient clinic to attend our combat veterans Tuesday and Thursday 6 o'clock group. I happened to have one more chair available in that group. I was happy to have him.

It is important to keep in mind that alcohol is a toxic substance. Abuse and even mild overuse of alcohol can have serious effects on a person's health:

- heart disease;
- high blood pressure;

- liver disease;

- impotence;

- nerve and brain damage;

- sleep problems;

- cancer; and/or

- damage to the stomach and kidneys.

Self-Examination for Alcohol Abuse

One of the most widely used measures for assessing alcohol abuse, the Michigan Alcohol Screening Test (MAST) is a questionnaire designed to provide a rapid and effective screening for lifetime alcohol-related problems and alcoholism (National Council on Alcoholism, 2021).

Carefully read each question and decide whether your answer is yes or no based on your behavior in the past twelve months. Choose the best answer that reflects how the statement applies to you or that reflects your feelings most of the time. Please note: This test will only be scored correctly if you answer every question. Check one response for each item.

1. Do you feel you are a normal drinker? ("Normal"—drink as much or less than most other people). Yes ___ No ___

2. Have you ever awakened the morning after some drinking the night before and found that you could not remember a part of the evening? Yes ___ No ___

3. Does any near relative or close friend ever worry or complain about your drinking. Yes ___ No ___

4. Can you stop drinking without difficulty after one or two drinks? Yes ___ No ___

5. Do you ever feel guilty about your drinking? Yes ___ No ___

6. Have you ever attended a meeting of Alcoholics Anonymous (AA)? Yes ___ No ___

7. Have you ever gotten into physical fights when drinking? Yes ___ No ___

8. Has drinking ever created problems between you and a near relative or close friend? Yes ___ No ___

9. Has any family member or close friend gone to any-one for help about your drinking? Yes ___ No ___

10. Have you ever lost friends because of your drinking? Yes ___ No ___

11. Have you ever gotten into trouble at work because of drinking? Yes ___ No ___

12. Have you ever lost a job because of drinking? Yes ___ No ___

13. Have you ever neglected your obligations, your family or your work for two or more days in a row because you were drinking? Yes ___ No ___

14. Do you drink before noon often? Yes ___ No ___

15. Have you ever been told you have liver trouble such as cirrhosis? Yes ___ No ___

16. After heavy drinking have you ever had delirium tremens (D.T.'s), severe shaking, visual or auditory(hearing) hallucinations? Yes ___ No ___

17. Have you ever gone to anyone for help about your drinking? Yes ___ No ___

18. Have you ever been hospitalized because of drinking? Yes ___ No ___

19. Has your drinking ever resulted in your being hospitalized in a psychiatric ward? Yes ___ No ___

20. Have you ever gone to any doctor, social worker, clergyman or mental health clinic for help with any emotional problem in which drinking was part of the problem? Yes ___ No ___

21. Have you been arrested more than once for driving under the influence of alcohol? Yes ___ No ___

22. Have you ever been arrested, even for a few hours, because of other behavior while drinking? Yes ___ No ___

Scoring

This self-test is scored by allocating one point to each yes answer—except for questions 1 and 4, where one point is allocated for each no answer—and totaling the responses.

Zero to two points: No Apparent Problem. Your answers suggest that you are in the normal range and at low risk of problem drinking.

Three to five points: Early to Middle Problem Drinker. Your answers suggest that you are at risk of problem drinking.

Six or more points: Problem Drinker. Your answers suggest that you are at risk of alcoholism.

This self-examination is meant only to be used as a first assessment, not as a diagnosis tool and should be used in consultation with a medical and/or mental health professional.

CHAPTER 13

# Painkiller Heaven

My clinical experience suggests that at least half of combat veteran callers who are suffering from PTSD are coming home attempting to transition into society with many PTSD signs and symptoms.

PTSD is extreme stress responses to a traumatic event that threatens the veteran's safety or makes the vet feel hopeless and helpless. Combat vets with PTSD may believe that they will never get over what happened or feel normal again, but with a timely intervention, a well-thought-out therapeutic treatment plan, and the support of loved ones, our returning warriors can overcome the symptoms, reduce the painful memories, and move on with their lives.

Vets need to know this: America does care about them! There are tens of thousands of Americans who have called or written letters to their State Representatives or other officials demanding an increase in veteran suicide prevention programs. Many veterans are emotionally distressed but say nothing to anyone.

Because veteran survivors have disturbing feelings when they feel stress or are reminded of their traumas, they often act as if they are in danger again. They might become overly concerned about staying safe in situations that are not truly perilous. For instance, a vet living in a safe neighborhood might still feel the necessity for an alarm system, double locks on the door, a locked fence, and a guard dog. Traumatized combat veterans often feel like they are in harm's way even when they are not, and they may be overly aggressive and lash out to protect themselves when there is no need. For example, a person who was attacked might be quick to yell at or hit someone who seems to be threatening. There are certain signs and symptoms to look for associated with PTSD and

TBI. Veterans exhibiting these signs should be encouraged to seek medical help immediately. Depression, anxiety, and panic attacks are all treatable mental health conditions. Call for help! At Appendix A of this book is a list of resources to help in these cases: telephone numbers, addresses, and contact information are provided.

PTSD and TBI are no small problems, according to Zoroya (2008), who reported that narcotic pain-relief prescriptions for injured U.S. troops had increased from 30,000 a month to 50,000 a month since the Iraq war began. Citing a leading Army pain expert, LTG David Fridovich, he questioned the drugs' potential abuse and addiction.

Lieutenant General David P. Fridovich was the Deputy Commander of the United States Special Operations Command (USSOCOM), MacDill Air Force Base, Florida. USSOCOM ensures the readiness of joint special operations forces and, he talks about dependency on pain meds following injuries associated with his post in special forces, and his rehab and recovery conducts operations worldwide. General Fridovich talks about dependency on painkillers following injuries.

Tony J. Cellino, Jr. felt the pinch that Zoya was reporting and that the general was describing. The 27-year-old, US Army Corporal, 10th Mountain Division, 3rd Brigade Combat Team was on a mission when he sustained injuries in a roadside bombing. He was rapidly deployed stateside to undergo surgery.

The story of decorated Army combat veteran, Corporal Tony J. Cellino, Jr., epitomizes the power of someone caring for his buddy's "wounded soul." I became aware of Tony's story through a call from one of his friends, Tim. Tim identified himself as a retired Marine and had called because he was concerned about the safety of his Army buddy. He wanted to read me a farewell note he had just received over the Internet from Tony. In the note, Tony stated that he had nothing more to live for, his wife and children had left him, he felt hopeless, emotionally numb, and detached from the Army, which no longer wanted him because of his PTSD and TBI concussion. The note put in plain words the combat veteran's feelings of rejection and discard and his loss of interest in activities and life in general. He wrote that he had already burned his service medals, commendations, and ribbons. Tim, alarmed, asked me what he should do? Tim did not know where Tony was located, just the fact he was out of town—he thought. When he called him, the voicemail message played. He only knew Tony's name, nothing more about his personal information. They had just recently become friends.

I asked Tim for the telephone number and Tony's full name. *We are running out of time*, I thought. The signs are all there for an impending suicide. He wrote a suicide letter, contacted his friend, burned his valuables, verbalized intent, and apparently had a plan, but we did not have all the details. I was aware of the need to act quickly, to take over the intervention. We did not have time to wait for the call to be traced for the location and police rescue. I had to call the veteran's cellular telephone number quickly!

I dialed the number. No one picked up, just an electronic digitized voice mail message. *Am I reaching the right phone? It isn't even a real human voice.* I was worried. "Stupid machine," I mumbled to myself. I hung up, leaving no message.

Up and out of my seat, I paced around my desk. I don't normally pace, but the tension was higher than normal. I moved over to the admin work area, peering in to see if there was any update. They reported no response yet from the cell phone company that was contacted to find the whereabouts of the vet's roaming cell number. Phone companies do have the ability to track cell phones.

The admin staff looked up at me as I poked my head in and said, "No word yet, Vic. We are working on it as fast as we can. We are at the mercy of the cell phone company but have contacted the police in the area as well as a heads-up in hope of getting some sort of lead." *We have nothing to go on*, I thought pensively. I felt I should not leave a message on Tony's phone. He might go into hiding if I did, and then we would lose our only possible contact.

I decided to wait a few more minutes. It was a tough few minutes. How many times could I look at the same clock on the wall, I mused. *Idiot! The clocks have nothing to do with anything. Come on, come on, Tony, where are you?* I brooded.

In a few minutes, I called Tony again. Again no pick up, but this time I felt I must say something into the recording to try and get through to speak to Tony. Time was slipping away. If I could facilitate my personal approach, heart-to-heart, buddy-to-buddy connection, we might have a chance to save his life. He was obviously feeling alienated. Tony had expressed feelings of rejection and abandonment. I knew if only I could talk with him, it would increase his chances for a rescue and getting him to a safe environment.

I felt in my very core that if I had but a minute to communicate to Tony, I had to express my true feelings of gratitude for his service to our country and demonstrate to him through my words, from one human being to another, that I cared. Then, I hoped he would respond to my plea for him to get some help.

Grabbing the telephone receiver, I decided to leave my message on the voice mail system: "Hello, Soldier. Oorah! My name is Vic, Thank you for serving our country, buddy. I am calling because Tim, a Marine friend of yours, called our clinic today and read me your e-mail suicide note. I hope we can talk this out, Tony. I don't want you to hurt yourself. You have too much life yet to live. I care about what happens to you right now, right here, okay?" I paused briefly, listening to the white noise in the background. Then, I continued, "A lot of people care that you served our great country, Tony. I am a former Marine. We are military comrades, buddies. You and I know what that means. We have a special relationship even though we have never met. I am watching your back, buddy We are here for you! Please call me back. I will wait for your call even if it takes all night. I want to talk to you, Tony. Please call, buddy." I gave him our clinic number. "Ask for me by name, Vic Montgomery."

I hung up the phone. Immediately, I alerted all the team that I was expecting an important return phone call, a possible veteran suicide in progress, needing a rescue. The wait was beginning to feel like time without end. I knew the feeling well. It is never easy when you really care about people and can unconditionally love a person even though you have never met him or her.

The call finally came in an hour or so later. I took it.

"Hello, Tony. What's going on, buddy? Thanks for calling me back. Your friend and I are worried about you." I left that statement dangling for a moment and waited.

"Thanks for calling me. Oorah!" Tony said in a quiet reserved manner. *Almost too reserved*, I thought and immediately contemplated that because of his calm, quiet demeanor he may have been medicated, self-medicating, already overdosing, cut, or something.

"Tony, are you still thinking about ending your life?" I asked him inquisitively.

"No reason to live. You probably already heard my story: no friends, kids are gone, no Corps, I'm a has-been." The proud warrior paused, cleared his throat, and said, "Corporal's all washed-up. Time to go."

He hesitated. I said nothing.

Then, he said, "Time to fall on my sword, Samurai warriors would say. Right, Vic?" he questioned as if he really wanted some relief from the sword idea.

I quickly responded, "No, that's not right, Tony. You do have a purpose in life and a reason to live—your children for one; children need their father. The grandkids will need their grandfather, too. It wouldn't be right to leave them. How old are the kids, Tony?" I asked, hoping to get him to talk by getting him involved answering questions. Very important!

"You don't really care how old my kids are, do you? Why do you care if I live or die? What am I to you?" The veteran's voice was quivering. I listened intently as Tony continued, "The Army didn't care who I was. They sent me packing, all because of a bump on my head. All I had was a bomb blast concussion. Now they're calling it TBI and PTSD. Now I have nothing to show for my years of service. My family moved out because I was acting strangely, moody, hard to live with, I guess. I can barely get a good night's sleep, even after 25 years, tossing and turning, experiencing flashbacks of the explosion in country. I remember feeling the growing danger in the weeks before the insurgents showed up. Snipers took potshots at our positions. After scrambling to locate survivors, handling body bags still bothers me. I dream of body parts. We had to match the body parts with the torsos and heads. I couldn't handle the nightmares and sleepless nights thrashing around, so I slept in another bed away from my wife. I knew we were in trouble when that happened several years ago. Things just started getting worse, slipping away. I am jumpy, quick tempered at times, and feel down in the dumps a lot. SOOO…they all left me like the Army left me or, should I say, booted me out." Tony took a deep, trembling breath, let it out, then went on, "Are you still on the line, Vic, or am I talking to myself, which I do a lot lately?"

"I am here. I have listened to everything you have said, and all I can say is wow, Tony. You have had a lot on your plate, buddy. Have you done anything to hurt yourself?

"Not yet."

"Tony, have you ever attempted suicide?"

"No," he responded bluntly.

"Tell me more about your suicidal thoughts. What's been happening in your life lately other than what you have just told me?" I asked frankly.

"My kids are 23 and 26. The last time I saw them was a year ago and then only for a brief visit. My family wants nothing to do with me. It seems no one understands what I have gone through. Vic, I am really hurting, down deep. Sometimes, I feel like I am suffocating. I wake up that way sometimes. I miss my kids. I have no reason for living without them. Nothing is going to change. I feel like I am in a dark, black hole in some other world, and it is lonely in that world, Vic, real lonely." He stopped talking. A bit of a frog in his throat, I figured.

"I am here for you, Tony. I won't leave you. I will stay on the line if you need, brother," I stated honestly.

Then, Tony unleashed a salvo of anxious expression, "It is like I am trapped and have no way of escape. I have had the same nightmare for years, seeing myself in a dark pit trying to crawl out, my fingers and nails worn to the bone bleeding. Then, I wake up, shaking and sweating. I spend my days sitting, staring at the walls in my house. I don't watch much television. I cancelled my cable when the kids moved out. I have been sleeping during the day and up at night most of the time. I am on disability for my medical condition. They say I have a traumatic brain injury. I get a check in the mail. It just barely gets me by. I see the VA doctor every month or so and get a couple of scripts and come home." The veteran warrior finally stopped for air.

"What is the medication for, Tony?" I asked.

"For depression and anxiety, panic attacks, all that stuff about PTSD, and, oh, I forgot to add my sleeping pills. I am a freaking pharmacy," Tony quipped. He continued in a serious tone, "Actually, Vic, you are the first person I have really had a straight-talk conversation with in many years, maybe ever, and to be honest it feels pretty good. I feel people really don't want to hear what I have to say or about my problems, so I just bottle it up inside. I never have talked much about my fears. I guard myself—tough guy, you know—stuffing my feelings is what I have always done. We guys have to hide 'em, or we're weak."

"So, now you have it all, Vic, which is why I want to stop this insanity. I can't take it another day. Too much, man, just too damn much." He paused for a fleeting moment. I, too, remained silent trying to process all of what I had just heard.

Then, Tony picked up where he left off. "That is when I e-mailed my suicide note to my vet buddy, Tim, and burned up all my Army stuff—medals and things."

"Tony, where are you calling from?" I asked inquisitively and an octave off-key. My voice cracks like this when I begin to get keyed up.

"I am on the Jersey shore, partner, on the boardwalk, having one last fling before I check out. Yeah, Vic, there is live music down here, rocking nightclubs and dance clubs where the beat never stops, they say, and, oh, yes, a mix of Irish pubs, traditional saloons, and sports bars you would not believe. Could you tell I'm an Irish, lad?" He did have a bit of an Irish accent. I didn't pick up on it until he mentioned it.

"Yes, Tony, now that you said something I believe you do have a slight accent," I said. And I added, "We are neighbors in the old country, lad. I am a Scotsman, and my family comes from the Scottish Highlands. In fact, Tony, I own a kilt."

"Yeah, but do you wear it? Hah," he laughed slightly and said, "That is a good one; small world really …," and he faded off for a moment.

I picked up the conversation. "Tony, I am glad to hear you are having a good time of it. Sounds like a nice getaway for you. What are your plans after the 'fling'? Will you be heading home?"

"Home?" he questioned. "A home I don't have? I am spending all my money, and when it is all gone, I am gone."

"What do you mean 'gone'?" I grappled for words.

"Yes, I have a plan. It is pretty simple, really. I have picked a nice spot overlooking the shore where I will park and end it. Poof! I will be gone, and no one will even care," he said with a timbre of tragedy in his voice.

"Where are you right now?" I asked with heightened interest.

"Right now, I am sitting in a motel room right near the boardwalk. Nice little place," he replied. "I am sipping on a bottle of warm ale, like they do in Ireland. Did you know, Vic, ale ferments best between 60 and 72 degrees Fahrenheit and therefore requires no special refrigeration or cooling."

"No, I did not know that, Tony," I said and then inquired, "What is the name of your motel?"

Abruptly, the phone went dead. "The phone went dead; his cell phone went dead," I ranted. I sprang from my chair and spun around, leaning on the balls of my feet, leaping forward, almost in one coordinated movement, and stepped out toward the admin room, repeating, "The phone died! I have lost him! I don't believe it! What do you have for a location on my caller?" I pleaded, "Tell me you have located his calling area."

"We know where he is, Vic, but not any more specifics than you already know. He is in a shore town in New Jersey. That's it. All we can get. The cell phone company said they can't get his GPS location," staff said downheartedly.

In agitated times like this, I have to pull myself together and focus. I began to ask myself relevant questions to weigh options. *What* are *the options here? How in the world do we find Tony?* We can't stop trying. At all costs, we must persist in the search for the suicidal veteran. *No warriors left behind!* I thought. Then, *when we locate him, how do I motivate him to come home and get help? I have already made it clear that I care about what happens to him, but the challenge as I see it right now is to encourage him to care enough about himself. Tony isn't thinking clearly. He is overwhelmed and confused. He has a wounded soul. Tony is brokenhearted. He lost his family; he lost friends in a roadside bomb; he lost his 10th Mountain Division Combat Team buddies; he has lost all hope.*

As a clinician I always must remind myself not to get caught up in my own emotional reaction. Sometimes, that is easier said than done. Therapists and counselors are taught to establish healthy boundaries, especially in times of emotional conflict. *When do I let go?* I asked myself. I got up from my desk and went out to walk the halls as I do when there is no resolution at hand and I am waiting for something to break. I resumed my thought. *Tony is going to kill himself when his last dollar is spent I thought, When will that be?*

I returned to my desk a few minutes later, spun my chair round, and sat down. Leaning forward, elbows planted on the desktop, I glanced down at my notes strewn around my desk. Many clinicians type their notes directly on the computer as they talk to the caller. Call me old-fashioned, but I write with pencil and on a yellow legal pad. That works just fine for me. As I was reading my notes, a thought came to me: I didn't know what method Tony was thinking about using for his suicide attempt. There was no mention of a weapon, knife, or gun. Ah, pills, I remembered. He has sleeping pills. *Tony what are you thinking? Where are you, buddy?* Still no word! I glanced up to look at the clock on the wall. *I have only a few hours left before I go home,* I thought. *What am I going to do? I can't leave him; I promised him I would stay on the line as long as it takes, but there is no open line now. His cell phone went silent.*

Tony did not call back that day. I called his friend and told him we had lost contact with him, that probably his cell phone battery went dead and maybe he did not have his battery charger with him. Or maybe he just didn't want to talk anymore. I told his friend we had the police looking for Tony, and we would do all that we could to bring him to safety.

We certainly don't win all the battles, trying to bring combat veterans in for mental health treatment, but fortunately, effective mental health treatments, such as those I pointed out earlier, are now available for many veterans with depression, anxiety, substance abuse, PTSD, and other war-trauma-related disorders. Unfortunately, most male and female warriors do not seek help. Many wrongly believe their symptoms are their own faults or are caused by personal weakness. They think if they try hard enough, they can overcome their problems by themselves, and they suffer unnecessarily.

In this case, Tony came back! A few days later I received the message that Tony had called his buddy a couple of days later and asked for my number at the clinic. Our staff who took his call told me Tony said he had changed his mind about ending his life and had returned home. He had called to see what he needed to do to get help. So, staff took the call and set up an appointment time to see me for an initial private consultation and group room #2 chair assignment.

How great a feeling is that! Some people would call it luck, or some would say it's not your time to go. I call it Heart-to-Heart Resuscitation...Oorah!

Signs and Symptoms of PTSD and TBI

The following are warning signs of either PTSD or TBI or both:

- Intrusive thoughts recalling the traumatic experience
- Nightmares
- Efforts to avoid anything that serves as either a reminder of the traumatic event or that triggers similar feelings

- Flat emotional response; little or no affect in facial expression
- Lack of motivation
- Depression
- Feelings of guilt (survivor's guilt is believing that somehow you were responsible for the death of comrades or civilians)
- Easily startled
- Insomnia
- Panic attacks
- Intrusive memories of the traumatic event
- Bad dreams about the traumatic event
- Flashbacks or a sense of reliving the event
- Feelings of intense distress when reminded of the trauma
- Physiological stress responses to reminders of the event (pounding heart, rapid breathing, nausea, muscle tension, sweating)
- Difficulty sleeping
- Outbursts of anger
- Difficulty concentrating or thinking clearly.

Warning Signs of Depression

Veterans should seek professional help if any of the following warning signs are severe or long-lasting

- • Excessive anxiety. This type of anxiety has no identifiable cause and is exaggerated for the situation. It can also manifest as a deep, continuing anxiety.
- Clinical depression. Severe depression is defined as persistent feelings of inadequacy, sadness, helplessness, hopelessness, undue pessimism, and loss of confidence as well as changes in behavior.
- Withdrawn. No longer enjoying the things that formally gave pleasure, including the company of loved ones and hobbies.
- A change in eating habits. Loss of appetite or overeating.
- Disturbances in sleep habits. Insomnia, an inability to stay asleep, or excessive sleeping.

- Low energy

- Chronic fatigue

- Ineffectiveness at school, work, or home.

- Decreased or no sexual interest.

- Isolation.

- Mood and behavior changes. Including gradual or abrupt or more frequent irregular changes between highs and lows. This does not include purposeful steps toward self-improvement.

- Physical symptoms. Includes headaches, nausea, tension, and unexplained pains.

- Views suicide as a solution (Strock, 2009)

Resources are available on the Internet

- Healthier You offers Ask the Medical Expert Archives (2000-2004) (http://www.healthieryou.com/medexpert/) and Ask the Mental Health Expert Archives (2001-2004) (http://www.health-ieryou.com/mhexpert/).

- Continuing Medical Education maintains a Health Directory of reference Websites (http://www.cmellc.com/resources/links.html).

- Mental health newsletter: Healthier You provides a register of Mental Health Mailing Lists (http://www.healthiery-ou.com/connect.html)

# CHAPTER 14

# Uppers and Downers

Marine Gunnery Sergeant James "Smitty" Smith had been a part of the 3/3 since 1983, when the 3rd Battalion, 3rd Marines deployed off the coast of Lebanon for several weeks during a particularly tense period in that civil war. He deployed again in 1990 as part of Operation Desert Shield and saw action at the Battle of Khafji and again during the liberation of Kuwait. In 2004, he once again deployed overseas in support of Operation Enduring Freedom in Afghanistan and in 2006 and 2007 to Iraq.

Smitty, 59-years-old and a retired veteran, was a distinguished Marine platoon leader. His fighting units were awarded Presidential Unit Citations for gallantry. He was the quintessence of esprit de corps. And he was addicted to uppers and downers.

Uppers give you extra energy, primarily by robbing your reserves. They keep you awake when your body really would rather be sleeping.

Downers send you to sleep and tend to lower your feelings and your sensitivity. They are therefore used to escape from the pains and problems of life.

Most people can identify with someone who is sad or mildly depressed because everyone has experienced these feelings before. PTSD depression, on the other hand, is a serious illness that involves a much deeper and more persistent depression with which few people can empathize. While someone who is sad may be cheered by a joke or able to "shake it off." this is not so with depression. A person suffering from major depression cannot will or wish it away.

My years of clinical experience have demonstrated that being depressed has nothing to do with personal weakness. I especially emphasize this fact with combat veterans. Most scientists in this field have generally known that developing knowledge of brain chemistry and findings from brain imaging studies reveal that changes in nerve pathways and brain chemicals called neurotransmitters can affect your moods and thoughts. These neurological changes may bubble up as symptoms of depression—including derailed sleep, suppressed appetite, agitation, exhaustion or apathy. In addition, I have found that genetic studies have shown that although no single gene prompts depression, a combination of genetic variations may heighten vulnerability to this disease.

Suicide is a frequent and sometimes lethal complication of depressive illness. Crisis intervention by trained interventionists or direct hospitalization should be sought immediately if the depressed veteran worsens or if the vet continues to talk about suicidal thoughts or threats of self-destruction. Counselors working with depressed veterans should refer them to professional help or have the vet call (possibly assisting with the call) the VA's suicide hotline at 1-800-273-TALK if the means of suicide are explicitly stated, if the veteran has lost his or her judgment to a point that he or she demonstrates a false sense of reality, if there is an obvious, even weak, nonlethal suicide attempt, or if the veteran's support system of family and friends is weak or unavailable.

Smitty, a 3-tour Army veteran of the war in Afghanistan, struggled with flashbacks and depression. "Asking for help is like letting my buddies down—very hard for me to do," he said. So, as a last resort before suicide and with Smitty's emotions beginning to erupt like an active volcano, I got his call at the clinic.

"I don't know what to do. My family is afraid of me and can't understand me. My best friends say I have changed. They don't come around to see me anymore. I can't face another day. I'm wasted."

"Smitty, what do you mean 'wasted'? Have you done anything to hurt yourself, buddy?" I questioned immediately.

His shaky voice continued, "You know. I spent so much time in Afghanistan, when I go out in my own backyard, I keep thinking someone is going to jump out from behind the bushes and zip me. I can't live like this. This is no way for a man to live: in fear. I am always looking over my shoulder, even walking down the street in my town. I'm wasted, man, burned up!"

"Smitty, are you thinking about suicide?" I asked directly.

Then, suddenly a loud voice began yelling in the background. It sounded like a woman's voice. She was talking so quickly the words were hard to make out. I heard, "Get help, Jim. You need help. Tell him."

As the voice came closer to the phone, I heard a rustling of the handset, and then the voice of the woman became clearer. "Here, give me the phone," I could make out amidst the commotion. "If you won't tell them, I will. Give me the phone, Jim. Hello, I am Jim's wife, Marsha. Is this the VA?" she asked dramatically and out of breath.

"No, I am a therapist at a local clinic. We often get overflow calls from the VA crisis lines. My name is Vic. How can I help?"

"Sir, my husband is having trouble, keeps telling me he doesn't want to live, and thinking about killing himself. He says, 'I'm going to waste myself and save you and the kids all the trouble and headaches of having to live with this madman.' I keep telling him to go to the VA and talk to a doctor, but he is stubborn as a rock and just won't do it. He says he can tough it out. He doesn't want to see any head doctors. I don't know which way to turn. Our kids are staying over at my sister's. I don't want to call the police." Marsha went on emotionally, "He has not had a day of peace since he returned home from that godforsaken place. You know, I don't know if he told you he went over there three times. Three times! I say God Bless America, but you'd think the military doesn't even care about our men. Three tours…just too much…too much for our boys. Each time he came back for a short time, it was like he was never here. And it seemed to get worse each time he came back. He mumbles under his breath about things I don't understand. Just the other day he started crying, sitting alone. I love him, Vic, but I feel helpless. Our marriage is crumbling around us. He gets real angry sometimes, throwing things. He put his fist through the closet door last week when he couldn't find something and accused me of hiding his camouflage jacket. He was drunk. He scares me even more when he drinks. I don't know what to do or how to act around him," she continued, unloading pent-up emotions. I listened, but I was wondering, *What is Jimmy doing? Where is he? Is he nearby listening to his wife fume?*

"And another thing," she said, still frantic. "What can I do? Where can I go for help? I don't know how to help my husband. He is slowly dying here, right here at home." She started crying.

"Marsha, we can help you and Jim…." Just then, Jim came back on the line.

"Hey, I heard what she said. It doesn't mean anything. She's all emotional right now. It isn't that bad around here; I'm okay, man. I just called you for a friend," Pete said fearlessly. *But I'm not buying that,* I thought.

"Smitty, you never did answer me—are you thinking about suicide?" I asked and then paused for the answer. "Yes or no, Pete?" I gripped the phone tighter.

Smitty apparently tried to put his hand over the phone mouthpiece, but I could still hear him say, "Marsha, go into the other room, and shut the door. I want to talk to this guy—alone! Please, trust me, I will handle this."

Faintly in the background, I heard a door slam. A moment passed. I waited.

"Okay, I have had those thoughts: killin' myself, getting it over with. I have this letter from the VA so I thought I would just call the number to find out what it was about." He paused.

"If you can, Smitty, tell me what you are thinking about, buddy. What has led you to thinking of ending your life? Was your wife right about the things she said? Was that accurate?" I asked, worried, hoping he would give me more information about his suicidal ideation.

"Oh, she overreacts some, but some of it is true. It has been hard for me and hard on them," his voice yielded. "I have these thoughts, you see. They don't seem to go away. I have nightmares about the battles with the Taliban, the insurgents. The noise of the AK-47s and rocket-propelled grenade launchers won't leave my head, and the faces of the Taliban fighters just keep coming and coming at me in my dreams. And the bodies, the blood squirting out of wound holes, the shuttering and jerking legs of the dead…it got so I lost all feelings. I just stuck to our mission, took care of business. I am a good soldier, lots of medals on my chest, good at what I did. It hardens a man, you know, especially the last tour. A good buddy of mine died. He was on my team. I saw him hit but couldn't get to him. I had his cover, but there were too many of them," he said sadly. "My wife doesn't understand…she can't." Smitty paused as if slipping into a zone. "Nobody can, unless you know what it is like having bullets flying by your head or are pulling the trigger or throwing the grenades. I don't want to talk anymore!" He abruptly stopped speaking.

"Smitty, I can get you and your family the help you need. There are Vet Centers and counseling for you and your family, outpatient or inpatient services. I have a clinic not far from you. There are PTSD and TBI clinics. Smitty, depression and anxiety are treatable conditions, successfully!" I explained. I felt the Sergeant was still listening on the line, but he said nothing. Hoping I had his attention, I continued.

"The line you called today has been started for you, Gunny, for veterans like you and your family, trying to reach out for help, but not knowing how to go about it. Smitty, will you let me help you?" I pleaded.

"Well, I see no harm in looking into it. What do I have to do?" he asked agreeably.

"Gunnery Sergeant Smith, I have an appointment slot open today, early afternoon at 1 p.m.; will you come in then? Or would 3 p.m., be better?."

"1 p.m. will work. What did you say your name was?"

"Vic Montgomery, Sergeant. Great! I look forward to seeing you in my office at 1 o'clock. Bye."

Smitty had three tours in the mountains and rugged terrain of Afghanistan. Lehrer (2009) quotes COL Elspeth Ritchie, a US Army psychologist, as saying, "Our research supports the more deployments that [a combat veteran has], the higher the likelihood of anxiety, depression and post-traumatic stress disorder."

Smitty's story shows how families are important resources for depressed returning veterans with PTSD. Family support can help prevent mental health problems. When problems do occur, it is often the family that recognizes something is wrong and helps the veteran to get care. Family and close friends often are the most pivotal advocates and can influence the veteran in getting to safety, and family members are important links to help veterans stay in treatment.

Resources for Families Seeking Help

*The National Center for PTSD*

The National Center for PTSD offers these reasons to seek help for PTSD:

- Early treatment is better.

- Symptoms of PTSD may get worse. Dealing with them as soon as possible might help stop them from getting worse in the future.

- Since PTSD symptoms can change family life from the vet's isolationist behavior, anger, even violence, getting help for PTSD can help improve your family life.

- PTSD can be related to other health problems. For example, a few studies have shown a relationship between PTSD and heart trouble. Getting help for PTSD, then, you could also improve physical health.

*Vet Center Program*

The Vet Centers Congress established the Vet Center Program in 1979 to help returning veterans readjust. The Department of Veteran Affairs maintains a website for families of veterans with PTSD and Vet Center resources, which explains:

> Vet Centers are community based and part of the U.S. Department of Veterans Affairs....The goal of the Vet Center program is to provide a broad range of counseling, outreach and referral services to eligible veterans in order to help them make a satisfying post-war readjustment to civilian life (Department of Veteran Affairs, 2007b).

Family members of all eligible veterans are also entitled to Vet Center services, including bereavement counseling.

The Vet Center offers readjustment counseling to veterans and family members of veterans who served in any combat zone and received a military campaign ribbon (Vietnam, Southwest Asia, OEF, OIF, etc.). The Vet Center defines readjustment counseling as a "wide range of services provided to combat veterans in the effort to make a satisfying transition from military to civilian life." Among the services included are "individual counseling, group counseling, marital and family counseling, bereavement counseling, medical referrals, assistance in applying for VA Benefits, employment counseling, guidance and referral, alcohol/drug assessments, information and referral to community resources, military sexual trauma counseling & referral, outreach and community education. "Readjustment counseling and other services are offered at Vet Centers for no cost. The Vet Center Directory is available on the Vet Center's website (http://www.vetcenter.va.gov/) or you can locate a Vet Center near you by looking in your local blue pages. Vet Center staff are available toll free during normal business hours at 1-800-905-4675(Eastern) and 1-866-496-8838 (Pacific) (Department of Veteran Affairs, 2007a).

*Supporting a Veteran with PTSD*

Melinda Smith, MA, Robert Segal, Ph.D., and Jeanne Segal, Ph.D. (2009) provide information for families helping veterans:

Be patient and understanding. A person with PTSD may need to talk about the traumatic event repeatedly. This is part of the healing process, so avoid the temptation to tell your loved one to stop rehashing the past and move on.

Try to anticipate and prepare for PTSD triggers.

Don't take the symptoms of PTSD personally. If your loved one seems distant, irritable or closed off, remember that this may not have anything to do with you or your relationship

Don't pressure your veteran into talking. It is very difficult for people with PTSD to talk about their traumatic experiences. For some, it can even make things worse.6

Here is some more information/help that can be given to families and partners of veterans with PTSD:

- Understand PTSD and flashbacks. Flashbacks can be equally as sudden, violent, and debilitating as epileptic seizures. The veteran may have experienced in the past or may be currently experiencing flashbacks and/or leg-thrashing nightmares that may cause him or her to sit up abruptly or leap out of bed. Loved ones of veterans need to be careful not to trigger a flashback by mistake. Two important ways to help with flashbacks are

    - knowing whether vet has them and

    - learning whether the vet finds comfort in the presence of others (typically, family) during them.

- For partners, don't ask about the details of a flashback since that might bring one on. Do ask if *you* have ever been particularly helpful in preventing or minimizing flashback effects. Build upon your natural ways of being supportive, and upon your partner's individual needs. Some partners want to be physically embraced. Others are made more anxious by a [person's] touch. Some partners do want to tell you details of terrifying memories, and they may want to repeat these details as a way of overcoming the threat. If it helps your partner, lend an ear. If you can't take it because you become too angry with a violent perpetrator or too over-whelmed with empathy, point that out, but be caring as you explain your limitation and do your best to find ways of increasing your emotional resilience so that you can be an effective listener (Ochburg, 2009).

- Veterans appreciate knowing that their loved ones are working to understand and cope with their PTSD, flashbacks and other symptoms. Therapy is helpful for both the veterans and their family members, but it may take several tries to find a good therapist to match the veteran's needs. Don't hesitate to change therapists if the veteran does not seem to be making progress, especially with overcoming flashbacks. If flashbacks are persistent, consider a mental health worker who uses re-exposure therapy. This technique guides the veteran through his or her traumatic memories and flashbacks in a controlled setting. Together, the mental health worker and veteran work through each memory to the end, eventually allowing the veteran to reconfigure his or her brain and develop the ability to remember at will. Trigger events are certain people, places, anniversary dates, smells or sounds that trigger reactions in veterans. These reminders are more sensations rather than memories. Mental images and sweaty palms are common reactions to trigger events. Talk calmly with your veteran about what his or her trigger events might be so both of you can identify situations that could be uncomfortable for your vet. Find out what triggers your veteran wants to avoid and help your vet do so without belittling him or her. Should your veteran choose to participate in a situation that possibly contains a trigger, make a plan together for removing the vet from the situation and trigger. Make sure the vet is involved in the process of planning an "escape"; having input in the process helps the veteran better manage triggers and feel more in control.

Partners of veterans with PTSD wonder how they can support their veterans when their veterans show little or no emotion; they seem emotionally numb and avoid being intimate. Many partners wonder if their veterans even still love them. Veterans need time to heal and cannot be rushed into emotions or intimacy. Encourage partners to continue to support their veteran and never blame him or her for the PTSD. Find out if they can accompany the veteran in therapy sessions or schedule sessions with the veteran's therapist for themselves. The veteran will appreciate support even if he or she is unable to express it.

Working in the field of crisis intervention and combat trauma, I often hear the question, "When is he or she going to get over it?" This is a natural and appropriate question but one that rarely has a definite answer. A veteran's therapist should be able to explain what is going well, what will take more time and the expected rate of recovery. It is not easy to overcome the emotional traumas of war, and the timeframe for recovery and healing will differ for each veteran (Ochburg, 2009).

# CHAPTER 15

# Medic Up!

I was dragging my butt this morning because we had an extra-long and emotionally tough night in group room 2 last night. So, I just slowly ambled over to the counter and picked up the file folder for my next appointment. After glancing at the paperwork, I thrust the folder up under my left arm, turned, and approached a veteran, who as in a wheelchair backed up against the wall of the far side of the waiting room. He was my 10 o'clock face-to-face after he called in for an appointment yesterday.

I noticed he was tatted heavily, arms and neck, and wearing pilot shades slid down on his nose as he stared back at me over the top of his sunglass rims with his bulging brownish eyes.

*Quite unapproachable* I thought. I immediately sat in the chair next to him so as not to tower over him but to be on an equal level, face-to-face. We bumped fists. I smiled, he scowled.

I said, "You must be Doc?"

"How did you guess?" he replied, staring at me with a halfhearted grin on his face as he grabbed the wheels of his wheelchair with his gloved hands. "And you must be Vic? Yes, my buddies do call me 'Doc.'"

"Well, yes, I am Vic. Welcome to our clinic, Doc Will you please join me back in my office so we can talk privately? I pointed the way to Doc as he began to swing his wheelchair in the direction of the hall.

We settled into my office down the hallway on the right. I closed the door. He chose to stay in his wheelchair, and I placed another office chair right in front of him and sat down. I offered him water.

The 66-year-old Army helicopter medic, Bill "Doc" Foreman served his country honorably with the 54th Medical Detachment, "Dust Off Missions," in 1965 in Chu Lai, Vietnam. During our initial phone conversation setting up todays' appointment, Doc shared that information and more.

"Doc, let me begin our talk today by saying I want you to know that I do care that you came in today. That took courage. I know that talking about the tough stuff, as we begin, will take a lot of trust between us. I know I must earn it. So, let me say this. I commit to you, Doc. I will not leave you or abandon you in your moment of need. I have your six, buddy. We are going to repair the brokenness and find out what and where the brokenness is. Oorah! I ask only one thing of you. Show me a willingness to change. That's it. And I will give you all the tools I have for your toolbox to make those changes happen. And one more thing…we have a group of combat vets you will be meeting tonight in group room #2 just down the hall from here that is part of your action plan."

Doc was listening to me, leaning over his legs and looking at his feet, wrapping his arms around his thighs and pulling up with pressure. I saw his ink-filled biceps strain and bulge against his legs.

He turned his head slightly, looking toward me. "I can do this, Vic. Let's get 'er done!"

"Doc, let's just talk. Tell me your story. Wherever you want to start." I said.

Doc began, "They gave me an M14 rifle and pistol, but, hell, under fire… trying to stop the bleeding of a wounded soldier …how the hell could I defend myself? I needed both hands in the wound. Shit, bullets were whistling by my head and mortars exploding all around. It was ugly. I can't get it out of my head. After all this time, I feel the fear. Our helicopter was bullet-riddled, and the bay was soaked with blood—one big nightmare, man. Guys were dying in my arms as body parts were missing. Who wouldn't need drugs to get through that? I had an unlimited supply of morphine."

Doc found a haven. Morphine is a narcotic pain reliever prescribed to treat moderate-to-severe pain, but the consequence also gives an abuser a false sense of well-being. When morphine is abused, an addiction can form very rapidly.

Survivor's guilt manifests as a combat veteran's mental condition when he or she perceives to have done wrong by surviving a traumatic event or several encounters. Survivor's guilt is a significant symptom of PTSD and needs to be identified and treated immediately. To learn how to recognize a veteran's battle with this vicious ailment and other dual diagnosis, a checklist of signs and symptoms of presenting problems can be found at the end of this chapter.

Doc began speaking with a surly voice. "It smelled of diesel; it smelled like death. It just engulfed me," he said, recalling the first days he had spent as a corpsman in Vietnam. Since returning, he had struggled with flashbacks, nightmares, PTSD, and depression.

"I have nightmares about those ponchos, slippery with blood. I seen bloody boots and the body bag zippers bleeding," he said in search of a reaction from me. "You tell me, counselor, how do I keep going? Why should I keep going? I am in my 50s, have had a stroke, and am trapped in my wheelchair. My legs don't work anymore. What's the use in living? Some days I feel guilty for being alive. I drink to numb my feelings and to pass out—to get some sleep. Most days, I don't want to wake up. You tell me—is that suicidal?"

"Doc, you are injured, partner, really hurt in the very fabric of your being. Your soul is wounded, buddy. I want to help you get through this feeling of helplessness," I said, making an urgent appeal.

With no response to my plea, the Vietnam warrior continued with his story, looking at his feet. I remember thinking at that moment, *how many years has Doc endured living like this, fighting with his hideous demons? I must help him; this is heartbreaking.*"

Doc continued, "In the months that followed, my company pushed against the North Vietnamese and the dense jungle undergrowth. We saw bodies lying infields …."

Doc explained, now speaking in a lower, more dejected tone, and with frustration in his voice. "I know firsthand the madness and violent cruelty of war in a way those in my family who have not experienced it cannot possibly know."

I responded, supporting him, "I hear you loud and clear, Doc."

He interrupted in dramatic fashion by sitting up in his chair and blurting out, "I can't get the images out of my mind, Vic!" The combat veteran was now shouting angrily, "My squad was put in charge of collecting our company's dead. And I was to patch up the wounded, triaging along the way. We were designated as the 'handling team.' When our team was notified, we carried the remains of our comrades to a collection site, downhill, downwind, and out of sight of the wounded and replacements." He hesitated. "I respectfully laid the bodies on tarps to help protect them from the weather." He paused again. I heard a slight but obvious sniffle.

"I'm listening, Doc," I interjected with a supporting timbre.

He continued, "And I...I took great care to help prevent the loss of their personal effects. I felt personally responsible to care for my fallen buddies. I was so angry when men of my unit just hung around, making rude remarks about the lifeless, 'killed-in-action' bodies by names like curly-heads, kinky-hairs, crew-cuts, or balding non-coms. I felt it was shameful," Doc declared sickeningly. "I felt sick and disgusted. The images of the dead, the faces when I was putting them in the bags, haunt me to this day. I am afraid to sleep some nights. I wake up wanting to puke. How can a man survive this nightmare for all these years?"

*Oh my! He wanted to keep talking, so I allowed him the room to express his pent-up feelings.*

This emotionally charged warrior cleared his throat and continued, "We then placed the KIA in the body bags by rolling the bags about halfway down the bodies and lifted both feet, after which we tied them together and pulled the green plastic bags down to their butts. Then, we lowered their feet, lifted the torsos, and pulled the bag up towards the shoulders and over their heads." Doc stopped talking abruptly. He sighed. And took a breath.

He hesitated for a couple of seconds before continuing. "Then, I closed the bags with a tie. I always made sure the zippers opened from the heads down. Me and my men then carried the bags to a truck, a cargo truck usually or whatever they had at the time to transport. It normally took three or four of us to lift one body bag onto a truck."

Doc paused, taking a breath. I sensed signs of a meltdown. I felt his anguish over what he had just told me. He painted vivid, compelling pictures as I listened intently to his story, a story I have heard before. Many emotionally scarred combat warriors had been given the difficult task of filling body bags and ponchos with the remains of their comrades, some stuffing the bags and poncho liners with only body parts.

There was silence. The room was still. I waited, watching Doc's body language. He sat quietly for the moment.

Doc, you obviously have been upset and burdened with these things you have told me for a long time, and you haven't ended your life or even tried. Right?"

"Right." Doc's head jerked backwards. "So, Vic, when were you going to ask me the question? Do I plan to kill myself? I can kill myself with guns, pills, and rope. In fact, I have a .38 Smith & Wesson at home on the table. I have a pharmacy of pills in my bedroom. As a matter of fact, I have a rope in the garage, and I know how to make a hangman's noose. So, what? Who the hell cares? I just can't live with all the pain and nightmares anymore. I have daytime flashbacks when I watch television. I see news special reports of the troops in Iraq, Syria, and Afghanistan, getting hit by roadside bombs, ambushes, snipers, and booby traps like in 'Nam. It brings back the tough times in country. I still can hear the mortar rounds of incoming that Charlie sent our way relentlessly, daily, body parts flying when the hits found their marks. And the yelling, 'Medic! Medic!' 'Doc, I'm hit! all around me still haunts me, Vic. I just can't take it. Everywhere I turn, the memories, and the sounds keep coming. You would think they would go away after decades, but not for me. I can't get rid of them." He paused. "I feel terrible most of the time when I sit here staring out at nothing, thinking that I made it out of country alive when many of my buddies did not. I ask myself, 'Why me?' A lot of good guys, Duke and Marshall, died over there. We went through boot together. A couple of buddies saved my skin, covered my back, and then were wasted minutes later. Now, I am trapped in my own cocoon, a wheelchair, most of the time not being able to get out of the house to my appointments or get groceries. But, oh, yes, big, bad Doc is still alive. How is this fair? This is no way to live—all these guilty feelings. I am getting too old for this shit. No future left for me," he concluded woefully.

Unresolved and unprocessed survivor's guilt can make recovery from PTSD and depression difficult. Therapeutic assistance is a valuable step for recovery and is important for persistent, intense guilt as well as other trauma symptoms that upset a survivor's life. As a combat veteran survivor, Doc needed to experience a renewed picture of his life. It was a matter of reframing his cognitive behavior. He needed help to change the negative thinking and unsatisfying behavior associated with depression and survivor's guilt while at the same time unlearning the behavioral patterns that contributed to his illness.

For Doc, it was extremely important to know, even if the rest of his life seemed insignificant to him, that many people were relieved that he was alive. He needed to reassess his past and to reassess what was valuable to him, reminding him that making the best of his life can be a tribute to his survival and to those who died in Vietnam.

I began H2HR with Doc on his very first appointment by immediately encouraging him to take the opportunity to reevaluate the meaning of his life. What was his spiritual condition, for example?

As an ordained minister, I firmly believe in the Holy Bible scriptures saying there is nothing more important than believing in a personal relationship with God. The Apostle Paul told Timothy,

It is equally important that Doc learn it is okay to take pleasure in being alive. It was as important for him to process and recognize, with therapeutic help, the reawakening of old wounds. His survival may have triggered old feelings of insignificance or dishonor. Surviving may have inflamed old messages that he received about not being worthy, about not measuring up as a combat medic, or about not counting. Doc had to learn to feel comfortable with the notion that it is good to survive and that it is in our nature to do so.

Doc suddenly interjected, "Hey, I have been ranting and raving for the last half hour, telling you my tales of doom and gloom, and I don't even know why I am unpacking all this."

"I know when you got back home from Vietnam, there was a lot of protesting going on, which was pretty ugly," I said. "You are a tough guy, Doc. Oorah! "

I remember thinking about the many articles and books I have read over the years after the War in Vietnam about the condemnation upon warriors return amplified the horror of his combat experience to result in an overwhelming degree of disgust. Staggering numbers of suicide among Vietnam veterans and the tragic number of homeless who are Vietnam vets, give evidence that something has occurred that is significantly and startlingly different from that occurring after World War II or in any other war our nation has ever encountered.

A former army Ranger and paratrooper, LTC Dave Grossman. who taught psychology at West Point and military science at Arkansas State University, writes in his bestseller book, *On Killing*, "What the epidemic of PTSD among veterans has caused is an increase of suicides, drug use, alcoholism, and divorce. Helping a veteran in such a situation involves encouraging him to share his experience" (1996, p. 349).

"I am here for you, Doc. We are very much behind our veterans, and I am here tonight to get you the help you need if you will let me," I said heart-to-heart.

"Are you a vet, Vic?" Doc asked, calming down.

"Yes, I am a former Marine rifleman, Vietnam, Doc. Oorah! And now I want to help you out of this situation you are in right now. You sound down in the dumps, buddy. I have your back, Doc!"

"But, Vic, I already see my doctors for my disability, heart, and stuff and have seen mental health doctors in the past. I have PTSD, they said, but I never really got caught up in the groups and treatment. I have tried to 'suck it up' myself. I have for years toughed it out. I don't like asking for help. Never have," Doc said deliberately. "My family doesn't have much to do with me. I don't make very good company. Not very patient and fire off at little things. Not many good friends, either. I am pretty much a loner and stuck in the house my mother left me when she passed on a few years ago."

He paused. "I really miss my mom."

Doc went silent. I could tell this was sensitive and protected territory. I didn't push for any more information. I sympathetically responded to his heartfelt statement about how close he was to his mother.

"I am here for you, buddy. Take as much time as you need." I waited, giving him the opportunity to speak again.

A few minutes went by as I shifted to a more comfortable position in my chair and glanced up at the clock on the wall while I was waiting for Doc to continue to open up,

Identifying symptoms is an important and vital step toward gaining an insightful understanding about depression. I have put together a rather simple "self-talk" test that may be helpful. Please keep in mind this is only a self-exam and is not intended to diagnosis depression or any other mental illnesses. That must be done by a doctor. A list of assistance numbers are located in Appendix A of this book.

---

SELF-TALK TEST

*Answer yes or no to each question.*

Do I have continuing thoughts about death or suicide?

Do I have thoughts or ideas and a plan to harm myself?

Have I tried to commit suicide in the past? Note: If you checked yes it is vital for your safety to contact the VA Suicide Prevention Hotline, 1-800-273-TALK(8255), for immediate assistance.

Do I feel guilty or useless?

Do I feel sad or irritable?

Have I lost interest in activities I used to take pleasure in?

Do I have trouble concentrating?

Am I eating much less than I usually do and have lost weight?

Am I eating much more than I usually do and have gained weight?

Am I sleeping much less than I usually do?

Am I sleeping more than I usually do?

Do I feel tired much of the time or more than usual?

Do I feel anxious and move around?

Self-Talk Test Total number of yes answers _____

If you have five or more yes answers, you may be experiencing major depression. Contact medical help immediately. If you checked fewer than five, you may be experiencing a mild form of depression. These are treatable conditions. In either case, please seek medical attention and advice as soon as you are able or call the hotline for assistance.

---

Doc said quietly, "She took care of me, Vic. I feel alone and empty now.

"Listen to me, Doc. Look at me! Look straight into my eyes."

Doc sat straight up looking forward.

"You care about people, which is why you took such good care of your fallen comrades over in the Nam. Our country needs good men like you to help youngsters coming back from Iraq and Afghanistan. The VA is always looking for volunteers to help give encouragement to warriors coming home. The vet centers around the country have counselors and groups you can be part of to share your experience, newfound strength, and hope. It is your time to shine, my man," I tried to encourage him. "I know it has been a longtime coming, but people now do care about Vietnam veterans, Doc. And many who were young hippie protesters back then now realize the mistakes made by not giving Vietnam vets a homecoming. Let us help you now. Your life has a purpose. It may be difficult for you to see it right now, but happiness is just around the corner for you, Doc. Brighter days are ahead, buddy."

There was silence. I waited. Doc was quiet. A few minutes went by.

I decided to break the silence. "Doc, the nightmares, flashbacks, and guilt can all be a thing of the past if you are willing to work with me. Begin today by going to group tonight in group room #2, right down the hall, our veterans' group. You don't have to live like this anymore, buddy. The group starts at 6 o'clock every Tuesday and Thursday for 90 minutes. Be a few minutes early for your first-time introduction. Okay?"

Doc nodded yes with thumbs up.

"Great! See you there. I lead the group."

"How about a dog?" I blurted out of nowhere. "You need a dog, Doc."

"What the hell are you talking about? A dog? What for?" he asked.

"That's the answer, buddy: a companion for you, a four-legged friend to keep you company, hang out with you, and look after you," I said in lifted spirits.

"What the hell? You are crazy, Vic! What am I going to do with a dog around my house?" Doc said frantically, caught by surprise.

"Have you ever owned a dog before?" I asked.

"Yeah...but a long time ago," Doc said. "My family had a Springer Spaniel. I haven't thought about that dog for a long time."

"What was her name?" I inquired.

"Lady," Doc replied, sounding proud to say her name.

"What happened to Lady, if I may ask?"

"We had to put her down after 18 years. She just grew old. Her back legs started giving out. I couldn't stand to see her in pain. I bought her when she was a pup," Doc shared, sounding a bit melancholy.

"Do you have room for a dog, Doc? A fenced yard?" I tried to get him interested.

Dr. Joan Esnayra, founder of the Psychiatric Service Dog Society, is in talks with the Walter Reed Army Medical Center about developing a program to train and place dogs with soldiers diagnosed with PTSD to try to help stem their problems based on research that shows that service dogs can help veterans with PTSD, sense oncoming panic attacks and depression and help overcome social isolation," which is a huge problem in suicidally depressed veterans (Shim, 2008).

"I have a yard," Doc replied, sounding a bit more interested. As for the rest of the story, we continued with quite a lengthy discussion about dogs and what great pets they make. We both shared great experiences and stories we had about them over the years.

"Well, Doc, we are out of time for today, buddy. Great getting to know you. Next face-to-face, next week, we will begin working on your treatment plan. See you later tonight for group. Six o'clock.

PTSD and Depression Signs and Symptoms Checklists

*Post-traumatic stress disorder (PTSD)*

PTSD may develop months or even years after the original war trauma and may include the following:

- Nightmares
- Flashbacks
- Efforts to avoid reminders of the traumatic event or triggers that evoke similar feelings
- Intrusive thoughts recalling the combat experience
- No self-motivation
- Depression (Refer to next checklist)
- Substance abuse: alcohol or other drugs, heavy drinking or drinking more than usual

- Feelings of guilt/survivor's guilt: from the false belief that one was somehow responsible for the loss of a comrade or multiple lives or civilian casualties in war
- Being easily startled
- Anger, easily agitated, irritability
- Lack of concentration
- Excessive awareness of possible danger, hyper-vigilant
- Trouble sleeping/insomnia (either not getting to sleep or waking up at all hours); the degree of depression, which only a doctor can determine, influences treatment.

*Depression*

Symptoms and indicators of depression, according to Ballas (2009), may include:

- Low tolerance to stress
- Low self-esteem
- Feelings of hopelessness and helplessness
- Agitation, restlessness and irritability
- Feelings of worthlessness, self-hate and inappropriate guilt
- Fatigue and lack of energy
- Behaviors such as "acting out" and being impulsive
- Sudden bursts of anger (not like before the war experience)
- Trouble sleeping or excessive sleeping
- Dramatic change in appetite, often with weight gain or loss
- Extreme difficulty concentrating
- Lack of pleasure from activities that normally made the veteran happy (prior to combat)
- Inactivity and withdrawal from usual activities
- History of alcohol or substance abuse
- Family history of depression, alcohol abuse or suicide
- Recurring thoughts of death or suicide.

# Conclusion

Roughly 16.5 million military veterans are living today in the United States of America. Approximately 1.6 million of those have served our great country boldly and loyally during the "thunder and lightning" of the Desert Storm ground invasion and air campaigns in 1991 on through to the conflicts in Iraq and Afghanistan. Tens of thousands are alive who served in wars and conflicts 50-60 years ago, including World War II, the Korean War, and the Vietnam War.

The need for healthcare isn't going away. It is mounting, especially because of the thousands of depressed, suicidal veterans who have been in hiding for too many years and are now seeking help.

Because of the pressure of the American people, especially many families living with troubled veterans and a more positive and proactive congress, more money and resources are being sent to the Department of Veterans Affairs to help these American heroes. We are beginning to see the results. The establishment of the National Veteran's Suicide Prevention Hotline is one example of action taken.

Another example is the huge effort to offer EF/OIF, Iraq, and Afghanistan combat veterans an accelerated assessment and evaluation process by the on-site crisis prevention coordinators at each of the 153 VA Medical Centers. These coordinators are psychologists, psychiatrists, therapists, medical doctors, and other highly trained healthcare team members who receive referrals directly from the National Hotline. The hotline's primary function and goal is to get suicidal veterans to safety, and the CPC will provide further referrals, treatment planning, and other treatment team support contacts at one of the Medical Centers.

I recall reading and hearing about the facts that our reservists and regular troops will continue to serve second, third and fourth tours in combat zones. The fact that men and women are sent into battle repeatedly raises many serious issues.

Many historians and seasoned military combat experts suggest for the first time in history, a sizable and growing number of U.S. combat troops are taking daily doses of antidepressants and sleeping pills to get sleep and calm nerves strained by repeated and lengthy tours.

It is important to be aware of these facts because well-documented statistics indicate that tens of thousands of combat veterans will be returning home suffering from a piling-on, adding layer after layer, tour after tour of PTSD symptoms. Many will find themselves struggling to transition back into society or becoming incapable of it altogether. This puts them at a higher risk of suicide.

Studies indicate that the probability for a combat warrior exhibiting signs of PTSD increases about 12 percent with each additional tour. Major depression and hopelessness, a significant sign in PTSD patients, have been implicated in 75 percent of all completed suicides. It is this hopelessness, constant bombardment of flashbacks and unrelenting nightmares with no end in sight that magnifies despair and substantially increases the risk of lethal behavior (Thompson, 2008).

Even if there is no suicide ideation, a vet may be experiencing other crises: unrelenting mental and physical pain, feelings of helplessness and hopelessness, substance abuse, addictions, and feeling out of control or in need of anger management and family counseling. Many disabled vets feel trapped with no escape. The pattern of veterans coming home but seldom reporting any mental health problems is also growing. These are just a few reasons to call for help and why we should care.

In this book, I have shared with you some personal stories and captured moments when vets or their family and friends called the hotline or came to outpatient clinics and emergency rooms, crying out for help. I have pointed out certain signs and symptoms that indicate when to ask for assistance. Seeking help is not a sign of weakness or something to be ashamed of. It is every veteran's right to seek help. As I've said previously and what is stated on that iconic poster, "It takes the courage and strength of a warrior to ask for help."

Feeling suicidal is a serious but treatable condition. Depression is a treatable disorder as well, with the proper care.

We have gone over how to recognize what defines a veteran's suicidal ideation, what signs to look for, and what to do they are discovered. Utilize the resource sections and checklists in this book to better recognize signs and symptoms of alcohol abuse and chemical dependency, PTSD, depression, and other emotional trauma.

I have shared how extremely distressing experiences cause severe emotional shock, which happens to many competent, robust, and rugged veterans. I sincerely hope I have conveyed the message and the facts that having such symptoms after serving in combat's traumatic events are not signs of personal weakness. Many formerly psychologically well-adjusted and physically healthy veterans develop PTSD because of the severe traumas to which they have been exposed.

Earlier in this book, I discussed how veterans who react to war traumas in such ways often feel depressed, out of control, and perhaps even feel they are losing their minds, but these physiological and psychological problems are treatable. The first important step to recovery is to educate combat warriors and their families so they can recognize the effects of emotional shock and know when and how to seek help. Suicidal thoughts can be troubling, especially when accompanied by depression, other mental health conditions, or alcohol or other drug abuse. The most important thing I hope to convey is that this situation demands immediate attention. These thoughts can indicate serious illness.

The up-close-and-personal stories and information in this book will, I hope, illustrate the impact depression and suicidal thoughts have had on the very souls of the veterans involved. The men and women veterans in this book are real people with whom I have talked and whom I have counseled. I hope reading of their experiences will those working with veterans to encourage them to plant their feet firmly on the ground, to put one foot in front of the other. To step forward. To reach out. To test the water of healing. They can do this. Their lives are very much worth saving.

# Appendix A

Veteran Support and Health Care

National Veterans Crisis Hotline

Do you or a veteran close to you have feelings of hopelessness or helplessness or depression? Are you stuck in a dark hole feeling there is no way out? Are you abusing drugs or drinking too much alcohol? Need help! Call toll-free the National Veterans Crisis Hotline: 1-800-273-TALK (8255) or 211 for immediate help anonymously or 988+1 for VA Crisis hotline.

Other Organizations

Here is information about some additional organizations and places you can get in touch with to find help. The following contact information was gathered from http://www.ptsdcombat.blogspot.com.

Gulf Coast VA Med Center Hot Line1-800-507-4571

Mighty Oak's Warrior Programs

33134 Magnolia Circle Unit 10

Magnolia, TX 77354

PO Box 1405 Montgomery, Texas 77356

Info@MightyOaksPrograms.org

Phone: (832) 521-7323

Miles Foundation1-877-570-0688

Military OneSource—DOD contracted1-800-342-9647 (24/7)

National Coalition for Homeless Vets1-800-VET-HELP

National Veterans Foundation Helpline1-888-777-4443 (M-F, 9-9 Pacific)

NY/NJ Veterans VA Nurses Helpline1-800-877-6976Suicide Help Onlinehttp://www.hopeline.comhttp://www.spanusa.org

Suicide Hotlines 1-888-649-13661-800-SUICIDE (784-2433)

Veteran Crisis Hotline with veteran-to-veteran counseling1-877-VET2VET(838-2838)

Veterans Affairs Suicide Prevention Hotline part of the National Suicide Prevention Lifeline1-800-273-TALK (8255)

Veterans of the Vietnam War1-800-843-8626

Wounded Soldier and Family Hotline1-800-984-8523.

National Service Organizations

Here is information collected from http://www.ptsdsupport.net on service groups that offer assistance during the process of filing a claim with the Department of Veterans Affairs. They will be the vet's representative before any review committee that will determine what rating of disability the vet will have if a claim is approved.

The American Legion National Veterans Affairs &Rehabilitation Division1608 K St., NW Washington, DC 20006Phone: 317-630-1200Toll-free: 1-800-433-3318 www.legion.org

AMVETS National Headquarters4647 Forbes Boulevard Lanham, MD 20706-4380Phone: 301-459-9600Toll-free: 1-877-726-8387Fax: 301-459-7924http://amvets.org/

Disabled American Veterans3725 Alexandria Pike Cold Springs, KY 41076Phone: 606-441-7300http://www.dav.org

Military Order of the Purple Heart of the U.S.A.5413-B Blacklick Road Springfield, VA 22151 Phone: 703-642-5360Fax: 703-642-2054www.purpleheart.org

Veterans of Foreign War National Headquarters406 West 34th Street Kansas City, Missouri 64111 Phone: 816-756-3390 Fax: 816-968-1149www.vfw.org

Vietnam Veterans of America 1224 M Street, N.W., Washington, DC 20005-5183 Phone: 202-628-2700Fax: 202-628-5880www.vva.org.

Veterans Integrated Service Networks (VISNs)

The Veterans Health Administration of the Department of Veterans Affairs is divided geographically into health system networks, called Veterans Integrated Service Networks (VISNs). Each medical center has points of contact to work with veterans from Operations Enduring Freedom and Iraqi Freedom. Further information on each network can be found at www.vacareers.va.gov/networks. cfm.VISN.

Combat Veteran Healthcare

The following information on healthcare eligibility, enrollment and women veterans is from the Web site of the Department of Veterans Affairs. Please refer to their Web site (www.va.gov) for the most up-to-date information.

Enhanced Eligibility for Health Care Benefits

The National Defense Authorization Act of 2008Veterans of Operation Enduring Freedom/Operation Iraqi Freedom (OEF/OIF).

Under the "Combat Veteran" authority, the Department of Veterans Affairs (VA) provides cost-free health care services and nursing home care for conditions possibly related to military service and enrollment in Priority Group 6, unless eligible for enrollment in a higher priority to:

- Currently enrolled veterans and new enrollees who were discharged from active duty on or after January 28, 2003, are eligible for the enhanced benefits, for 5 years post discharge

- Veterans discharged from active duty before January 28, 2003, who apply for enrollment on or after January 28, 2008, are eligible for the enhanced benefit until January 27, 2011.

Who's Eligible? Veterans, including activated Reservists and members of the National Guard, are eligible if they served on active duty in a theater of combat operations after November 11, 1998, and have been discharged under other than dishonorable conditions.

Documentation Used to Determine Service in a Theater of Combat Operations

- military service documentation that reflects service and the combat theater; receipt of combat service medals; and/or
- receipt of eminent danger or hostile fire pay or tax benefits.

Health Benefits Under The "Combat Veteran" Authority

- Cost-free care and medications provided for conditions potentially related to combat service.
- Enrollment in Priority Group 6 unless eligible for enrollment in a higher priority group.
- Full access to the VA's Medical Benefits Package

What happens After the Enhanced Eligibility Period Expires? Veterans who enroll with VA under this authority will continue to be enrolled even after their enhanced eligibility period ends. At the end of their enhanced eligibility period, veterans enrolled in Priority Group 6 may be shifted to Priority Group 7 or 8, depending on their income level, and required to make applicable co-pays.

What About Combat Veterans Who Do Not Enroll During Their Enhanced Authority Period? For those veterans who do not enroll during their enhanced eligibility period, eligibility for enrollment and subsequent care is based on other factors such as: a compensable service-connected disability, VA pension status, catastrophic disability determination, or the veteran's financial circumstances. IMPORTANT: For this reason, combat veterans are strongly encouraged to apply for enrollment within their enhanced eligibility period, even if no medical care is currently needed.

Enrollment Guidelines

- Currently enrolled combat veterans will have their enhancement enrollment period automatically extended to 5 years from their most recent date of discharge.
- New enrollees discharged from active duty on or after January 28, 2008 are eligible for this enhanced enrollment health benefit for 5 years. after the date of their most recent discharge from active duty.

- Combat veterans who never enrolled and were discharged from active duty between November 11, 1998 and January 27, 2003 may apply for this enhanced enrollment opportunity through January 27, 2011.

- Combat veterans who applied for enrollment after January 16,

Combat veterans who applied for enrollment after January 16, 2003, but were not accepted for enrollment based on the application being outside the previous post-discharge two year window will be automatically reviewed and notified of the enrollment decision under this new authority: National Defense Authorization Act of 2008.

Additional Information Regarding Combat Veteran Benefits

Additional information is available at your nearest VA facility or Veterans Service Center and by calling toll-free 1-800-827-1000 or 1-877-222-8387

National Resource Directory Offers Veterans One-Stop Info and Access to Myriad Health, Employment Services

The Department of Defense launched the National Resource Directory, a collaborative effort between the departments of Defense, Labor and Veterans Affairs. The directory is a Web-based network of care coordinators, providers and support partners with resources for wounded, ill and injured service members, veterans, their families, families of the fallen and those who support them. "The directory is the visible demonstration of our national will and commitment to make the journey from 'survive to thrive' a reality for those who have given so much. As new links are added each day by providers and partners, coverage from coast to coast will grow even greater ensuring that no part of that journey will ever be made alone," said Lynda C. Davis, Ph.D., deputy undersecretary of defense for military community and family policy. Located at www.nationalresourcedirectory.org, the directory offers more than 10,000 medical and non-medical services and resources to help servicemembers and veterans achieve personal and professional goals along their journey from recovery through rehabilitation to community reintegration.

Disabled Veterans

Veterans who are 50 percent or more disabled from service-connected conditions, unemployable due to service-connected conditions, or receiving care for a service-connected disability receive priority in scheduling of hospital or outpatient medical appointments.

How do I get my disability compensation claim reevaluated? You may request a reevaluation of your claim anytime that you believe your condition has changed or worsened. Submit the request to reopen or reevaluate your claim to the VA Regional Office in either letter or statement form or on VA Form21-4138 (Statement in Support of Claim): http://www.vba.va.gov/pubs/forms/21-4138x.pdf). Request should include the following information:

- Name
- Claim number or Social Security Number
- Day and evening contact information• Current address• Statement explaining change requested
- Any new and pertinent medical evidence that supports your request.

Homeless Veterans

VA offers a wide array of special programs and initiatives specifically designed to help homeless veterans live as self-sufficiently and independently as possible. In fact, VA is the only Federal agency that provides substantial hands-on assistance directly to homeless persons. Although limited to veterans and their dependents, VA's major homeless-specific programs constitute the largest integrated network of homeless treatment and assistance services in the country. VA's specialized homeless veterans' treatment programs have grown and developed since they were first authorized in 1987. The programs strive to offer a continuum of services that include:

- Aggressive outreach to those veterans living on streets and in shelters who otherwise would not seek assistance.
- Clinical assessment and referral to needed medical treatment for physical and psychiatric disorders, including substance abuse.
- Long-term sheltered transitional assistance, case management and rehabilitation.
- Employment assistance and linkage with available income supports; and
- Supported permanent housing. How do I contact a coordinator for options for women veterans who are home-less with children? Contact the local VA homeless coordinator (or point of contact), Social Work Services department or Women Veterans Coordinator at your local VAMC. There are homeless women veterans and homeless women

veterans with children pilot programs located at eleven designated VA facilities as well, and the Women Veterans Coordinator can discuss what options are available in your area.

Women in Uniform

The Department of Veterans Affairs has experienced a number of successes for women veterans. These successes include:

- Legislative gains in the areas of military sexual trauma, homeless women veterans programs, special monthly compensation for women veterans who lose a breast as a result of a service-connected disability (final regulation effective March 18, 2002), maternity and infertility services and studies indicating negative reproductive outcomes in women veterans who served in-country in Viet Nam.

- Receipt of the 2000 Wyeth-Ayerst Bronze HERA Award in recognition of Veterans Health Administration's demonstrated leadership in women health.

- Guidance in the assessment and treatment of infertility in both women and men.

- Women Veteran Program Managers (WVPM) at every VA Medical Center and Women Veterans Coordinators at every Regional Office.

- Increased coordination and expert consultation through the appointment of a Lead Women Veteran Program Managers in all twenty-one networks

- Establishment of specialized and frequently separate women's health clinics in nearly two-thirds of VA medical centers, as well as women's health providers or teams within primary care practices.

  - Migration of Women Veterans Health and Military Sexual Trauma Software with Computerized Patient Record System.

  - Gains in the number of corrective actions taken relative to women veterans 'privacy deficiencies

- In April 2002, the Women's Health Program sponsored a national women veterans coordinators (WVCs) conference bringing together WVCs nation-wide from both Veterans Health Administration and Veterans Benefits Administration to discuss women veterans issues and network so that services to women veterans with benefits and health issues can now be accomplished more smoothly.

For more information contact the Center for Women Veterans, 202-273-6193.

Where are the special PTSD treatment centers for women? Women Veteran Stress Disorder Treatment Programs have been established at the following VA sites (see the VISN listing for telephone numbers): Boston, MA Brecksville, OH Loma Linda, CA New Orleans, LA

Where can I get Military Sexual Trauma treatment? You may enroll and receive counseling and treatment for any emotional or physical condition experienced, as a result of sexual trauma experienced while on active duty, at any VA health care facility or Rehabilitation Counseling Center (Vet Center) in the continental United States without regard for your service-connected rating or length of military service through December 31, 2004.

Where can I get inpatient psychiatric care as a woman veteran? Most VA Medical Centers have inpatient mental health programs. Contact your VA Primary Care Provider or the local Mental Health Program office for assistance. If you already have a therapist and need inpatient care, please dis-cuss your concerns with your therapist. If you have urgent or emergency needs, you can contact your local VA health care facility telephone care program or urgent care clinic.

Where are the designated Clinical Programs of Excellence in Women's Health?

- Women Veterans Health Care Program, Alexandria, VA
- VAMC Women Veterans Comprehensive Health, Durham, NC
- VAMC Women Veterans Health Program, Boston, MA
- VAMC, VA
- Veterans Health Program, Bay Pines, FL
- VA Healthcare System Women Veterans Health Program, Pittsburgh, PA
- South Texas Veterans Health Care System, South Texas-Arlington, TX

Pet Therapy

Pet Therapy Canine Helpers for the Handicapped, Inc. is a non-profit organization dedicated to training dogs to assist individuals with disabilities to lead more independent and secure lives. This organization provides custom-trained assistance service dogs for mobility, hearing impaired, PTSD and therapy. Canine Helpers for the Handicapped, Inc.5699 Ridge Road (RT. 104) Lockport, New York 14094716-433-4035/ Fax 716-439-0822 Email: CHHDogs@aol.com; Web site: http://www.caninehelpers.org/

# Appendix B

Veteran Resources

Alexander, Bevin. (1986). *Korea: The First War We Lost*. New York: Hippocrene Books.

American Psychiatric Association. (2000). *Diagnostic and Statistical Manual of Mental Disorders: DSM-IV-TR,4thed., Text Revision*. Washington, D.C.: American Psychiatric Association Publications.

Anon. (2023). Addiction Medicine, http://www.Addiction-medicine.org.The America's Intelligence Wire: Desert Storm, www.navy.mil.

Anon. (2023). "How to Talk to a Suicidal Friend." Downloaded from http://www.ehow.com/how_2071390_talksuicidalfriend.html?ref=fuel&utm_source=yahoo&utm_medium=ssp&utm_campaign=yssp_art.

Aphrodite, Matsakis,. (1991). *I Can't Get Over It: A Handbook for Trauma Survivors*. Oakland, CA: New Harbinger Publications, Inc., pp. 228-337.

Clair, Clay. *The Forgotten War*. New York: Time Books, 1987.

Craigie, Jr. Frederick C. (2020). *Weekly Soul: Fifty-two Meditations on Meaningful, Joyful, and Peaceful Living*. Hollister, CA: MSI Press LLC. The meditations begin with thought-provoking quotations from a range of people-writers, journalists, theologians, musicians and artists, activists—and touch on themes of Miracles, Aliveness, Purpose, Laughter and Joy, Presence/Mindfulness, Activism, Acceptance, Gratitude, Forgiveness, Creativity, Civility, and Hope.

Dawe, Brice. (2023). "Analysis of 'Homecoming.'" Downloaded from http://literatureclassics.com/essays/408/.

Everyday Health.http://www.everydayhealth.com/depression/understanding/what-is-depres-sion.aspx.

Fibromyalgia Network. http://www.fmnetnews.com.F

Fort Campbell Crisis Assistance. http://www.campbell.army.mil/crisis/index.html.

Goulden, Joseph. (1982). *Korea: The Untold Story of the War.* New York: Time Books.

Hall, Calvin S., & Lindzey, Garnder. (1970). *Theories of Personality.* New York: Wiley and Sons, Inc.

Halliday, Jon, & Cummings, Bruce. (1988). *Korea: The Unknown War.* New York: Pantheon Books.

Harvard Health Publications. "What Is Depression?" Harvard Health Publications Special Health Report.

Hastings, Max. (1987). *The Korean War.* New York: Simon & Shuster.

Hedrick, Susan, et al. (2003). "Resident Outcomes of Medicaid-Funded Community Residential Care." *Gerontologist 43*: 473-482.

Hedrick, Susan, et al. (2007). "Characteristics of Residents and Providers in the Assisted Living Pilot Program." *Gerontologist 47*: 365-77.

Integrative Medicine Communications. (2023). "Post-Traumatic Stress Disorder." *Integrative Medicine Access.* Downloaded from http://www.gardenoflight.net/Site2/Research_Center/library/ConsConditions/Print/PosttraumaticStressDisordercc.html.

Kerr, Jennifer C. (May 2007). "Veterans' Group Emphasizes Suicide Risks," *SFGate.* Downloaded from http://www.sfgate.com/cgi-bin/article.cgi?f=/n/a/2007/05/28/national/w135433D60.DTL.

Kim, Chum-kon. (1973). *The Korean War 1950-53.* Seoul: Kwangmyong Publishing Company.

Lowary, Jake. (January 2008). "New post clinics to fight dual threat: PTSD, TBI." *Veterans for America.* Downloaded from http://www.veteransforamerica.org/2008/01/25/new-post-clinics-to-fight-dual-threat-ptsd-tbi/.

Meagher, Ilona, ed. (September 15, 2008). "OEF/OIF Veteran Suicide Toll: Nearly 15% of Overall U.S. Military Casualties Result from Suicide." *PTSD Combat: Winning the War Within*. Downloaded from http://ptsdcombat. blogspot.com/2008/09/oefoif-veteran-suicide-toll-15-of.html.

MacDonald, Callum A. Korea: The War before Vietnam. New York: Macmillan,1986

Matloff, Maurice, ed. American Military History. Washington: Center of Military History, 1969.

McFall, E. Everett. (2007). *I Can Still Hear Their Cries: Even In My Sleep*. Denver: Outskirts Press.

Meagher, Ilona, ed. PTSD Combat: Winning the War Within. Http:// ptsdcombat.blogspot.com.Mundell, E.J. "Younger Veteran at Greater Suicide Risk." U.S. News and World Report. 10 October 2007. http://health.usnews. com/usnews/health/health-day/071030/younger-veterans-at-greater-suicide-risk.htm.

Paschall, Rod. 1995. *Witness to War, Korea*. New York: Perigee.

Pratt, Sherman W. (1992). *Decisive Battles of the Korean War*. New York: Vantage Press.

Principi A.J. (November 23, 2004). Letter to Arlen Specter, Chairman, Committee on Veterans' Affairs, United States Senate.

Prolastin. (2023). "Managing Stress." *Talecris Biotherapeutics, Inc.* Downloaded from http://www.pro-lastin.com/4.5.0_cons_stress.aspx.

PTSD Support Services. http://www.ptsdsupport.net.

Reinberg, Steven. (January 12, 2009). "With Depression Vets Face Higher Suicide Risk." *Health Day*. Downloaded from http://www.healthday.com/ Article.asp?AID=622964.

Ridgway, Matthew B. 1967. *The Korean War*. New York: Doubleday.

Russ, Martin. (1957). *The Last Parallel*. New York: Kensington.

Segal, Jeanne, ed. (2023). "Help Guide." Downloaded from http://www. helpguide.org/.

Stokesbury, James L. (1988). *A Short History of the Korean War*. New York: William Morrow & Co.

Summers, Harry G., Jr. (1990). *Korean War Almanac*. New York: Facts on File.

The *New York Times*. (2023). *Health Guide*. Downloaded from http://health. nytimes.com/health/guides/disease/suicide-and-suicidal-behavior/overview. html?inline=nyt-classifier.CMPMedica, LLC

Times. http://www.timesonline.co.uk/tol/news/world/us_and_americas/article2873622

Van Wagner, Kendra. (2023). "Color Psychology: How Colors Impact Moods, Feelings, and Behaviors." *About.com*. Downloaded from http://psychology. about.com/od/sensationand-perception/a/colorpsych.htm.

Veteran Internet References. (May 21, 2009). "An Abstract Bibliography: Journal Articles." *Diagnosis and Treatment of Combat Related Post-Traumatic Stress Disorder* (p. 226). Downloaded from http://www.crdamc.amedd.army. mil/library_med/PTSD_Bibliography.pdf.Veterans(001-236).qxp.

Victoroff, Victor. (1983). *The Suicidal Patient: Recognition, Intervention, Management*. Oradell, NJ: Medical Economics Books.

Walter Reed Army Institute of Research. (2023). "Concussions Occurring Among Our Soldiers Deployed in Iraq," Downloaded from http://wrair-www. army.mil/images/MildTBI.pdf.

Waterfront Media, Inc. (2023). "Depression Checklist." *Everyday Health Network*. Downloaded from http://www.everydayhealth.com/publicsite/index. aspx?puid=0512F6BA-8101-4877-B11D-3E99973800D4&p=2.

Wikipedia. (2023). *PTSD*. Downloaded from http://www.crdamc.amedd. army.mil/library_med/PTSD

Wilkerson, Dave. (1982). *Have You Felt Like Giving Up Lately?* Grand Rapids, MI: Revell.

Witt, P.H., Greenfield, D. P., & Steinberg, J. (1993). "Evaluation and Treatment of Post-Traumatic Stress Disorder. *New Jersey Medicine 90 no. 6*: 464-467.

Wood, Starr A. (2023). "Crisis Intervention." Downloaded from http://www. albany.edu/~sawood/crisis%20intervention.htm.

Zivin, Kara, H., Kim, Myra, McCarthy, John F., Austin, Karen L., Hoggatt, Katherine J., Walters, Heather H., & Valenstein, Marcia. (2007). "Suicide Mortality Among Individuals Receiving Treatment for Depression in the Veterans Affairs Health System: Associations with Patient and Treatment Setting Characteristics." *American Journal of Public Health 97no. 12*: 2193-8.

# References

Armstrong, Keith, Suzanne Best, Paula Domenici and Bob Dole. *Courage After Fire: Coping Strategies for Troops Returning from Iraq and Afghanistan and Their Families*. Berkeley, CA: Ulysses Press, 2006.

Baldwin, T. (November 2007). America suffers an epidemic of suicides among traumatized army veterans. *Times Online*.

Ballas, Paul. (January 2009). "Medical Encyclopedia: Depression." *Medline Plus*. Downloaded from http://wwwils.nlm.nih.gov/medlineplus/ency/article/003213.htm.

Boom, Corrie Ten. (1953). *Amazing Love: True Stories of the Power of Forgiveness*. Grand Rapids, Michigan: Baker Book House.

Carlson Eve B., & Ruzek, Josef. (2004). "Effects of Traumatic Experiences: A National Center for PTSD Fact Sheet." *National Center for Post-Traumatic Stress Disorder*. Downloaded from http://www.ncptsd.org/facts/general/fs_effects.html(accessed 2009) (site now discontinued)

Carroll, Jill. (July 2008). When the war comes back home. *The Christian Science Monitor*. Downloaded from http://www.csmonitor.com/2008/0712/p02s01-usmi.html.

Coleman, Penny. (2006). *Flashback: Posttraumatic Stress Disorder, Suicide, and the Lessons of War*. Boston: Beacon Press.

Department of Veterans Affairs. (October 2007a.) "Services—Vet Center." Downloaded from  http://www.vetcenter.va.gov/Vet_Center_Services.asp

Department of Veterans Affairs. (October 2007b). "Who We Are—Vet Center," Downloaded from http://www.vetcenter.va.gov/About_US.asp.

Emmite, Debra, & Swierzewskit III, Stanley J. eds. (March 2008). "Alcohol Abuse: Treatment, Prognosis." *Healthcommunities.com, Inc.* Downloaded from http://www.mentalhealthchannel.net/alcohol/treatment.shtml.

Global Security (2006). "Fallujah." Downloaded from http://www.globalsecurity.org/military/world/iraq/fallujah.htm.

Grossman, D. (1996). *On killing: The Psychological Cost of Learning to Kill in War and Society* New York: Back Bay Books.

Metzger, D. (2002). *Entering the Ghost River.* Topanga, CA: Hand to Hand.

Holmstedt, Kirsten. (2007). *Band of Sisters: American Women at War in Iraq.* Mechanicsburg, PA: Stackpole Books.

Johnson, Spencer. (1992). *The Precious Present.* New York: Doubleday.

Lehrer, Jim. (January 29, 2009). "The War Briefing." *News Hour, PBS, MacNeil/Lehrer Productions.* Downloaded from http://www.pbs.org/newshour/bb/health/jan-june09/suicides_01-29.html.

Mandino, Og. (1985). *The Greatest Salesman in the World.* Hollywood, FL: Fredrick Fell Publishers, Inc.

Matsakis, Aphrodite. (2007). *Back from the Front: Combat Trauma, Love, and the Family.* Baltimore, MD: Sidran Institute Press.

Meagher, I., ed. (September 15, 2008). "OEF/OIF veteran suicide toll: Nearly 15% of overall U.S. military casualties result from suicide." *PTSD Combat: Winning the War Within.* Downloaded from http://ptsdcombat.blogspot.com/2008/09/oefoif-veteran-suicide-toll-15-of.html.

Miller, Michael Craig, ed. (2008). *Understanding Depression.* Cambridge, MA: Harvard Health Publications.

Moore, Pamela R. (2004). *Life Lessons from the Hiding Place: Discovering the Heart of Corrie Ten Boom.* Grand Rapids, MI: Chosen Books.

National Center for PTSD. 2023. "What can I do if I think I have PTSD?" Downloaded from http://www.ncptsd.va.gov/ncmain/ncdocs/fact_shts/fs_what_can_i_do.htm.

National Council on Alcoholism. 2021. MAST Self-Test. Downloaded from www.thenationalcouncil.org.

NBC News. (May 19, 2009). US Military: Heavily Armed and Medicated. Downloaded from https://www.nbcnews.con/health/health-news/u-s-military-heavily-armed-medicated-flna1CMeagher9453648.

Ochberg, Frank. (February 2009). :Partners With PTSD." *Gift from Within*. Downloaded from http://www.giftfromwithin.org/html/partners.html.

O'Donnell, Patrick K. (2004). *We Were One: Shoulder to Shoulder with the Marines Who Took Fallujah*. Cambridge, MA: Da Capo Press.

Olenchek, Christina. (November/December 2008). "Dialectical Behavior Therapy—Treating Borderline Personality Disorder." *Social Work Today*. Downloaded from http://www.socialworktoday.com/archive/102708p22.shtml.

Rogers, C. R. (1957). "The Necessary and Sufficient Conditions of Therapeutic Personality Change. *Journal of Consult Psychol*ogy 21(2):95-103.

Rogers, C. (1959). "A Theory of Therapy, Personality and Interpersonal Relationships As Developed in the Client-centered Framework. In (ed.) S. Koch, *Psychology: A Study of a Science. Vol. 3: Formulations of the Person and the Social Context*. New York: McGraw Hill.

Rogers, C. (1961). *On Becoming a Person*. Boston: Houghton-Mifflin.

Schirldi, Glen R. (2000). *Posttraumatic Disorder Sourcebook: A Guide to Healing. Recovery, and Growth*. Lincolnwood, IL.: Lowell House.

Shim, Joan. (January 2008). "Dogs chase nightmares of war away." *CNN* Downloaded from http://www.cnn.com/2008/LIVING/personal/01/29/dogs.veterans/index.html (accessed 2009).

Smith, Melinda, Segal, Robert, & Segal, Jeanne. (November 2008). "Post-Traumatic Stress Disorder (PTSD): Symptoms, Treatment, and Self-Help." *Help Guide*. Downloaded from http://www.helpguide.org/mental/post_151traumatic_stress_disorder_symp-toms_treatment.htm.

Standal, S. (1954). *The Need for Positive Regard: A Contribution to Client-centred Theory*. Unpublished PhD. thesis, University of Chicago.

Strock, Margaret Strock, ed. (2009). "You Are Not Alone." *Healthier You*. http://www.healthieryou.com/alone.html.

Thompson, Mark. (June 5, 2008). America's Medicated Army. *Time*. Downloaded from http://www.time.com/time/nation/article/0,8599,1811858,00.html

Tick, Edward. (2005). *War and the Soul: Healing Our Nation's Veterans from Post-Traumatic Stress Disorder*. Wheaton, IL: Quest Books.

Tull, Matthew. (September 2007). "Military Sexual Trauma and PTSD among Female Veterans." *About.com*. Downloaded from http://ptsd.about.com/od/causesanddevelop-ment/a/PTSDandMST.htm.

Tull, Matthew. (February 2009). "Military Sexual Trauma and the Iraq War." *About.com*. Downloaded from http://ptsd.about.com/od/ptsdandthemilitary/a/MSTOFE-FOIF.htm.

Valles, Sean. (June 2007). "US Trying Hard to Provide Proper Treatment for Wounded Soldiers." *Bio-Medicine*. Downloaded from http://www.bio-medicine.org/medi-cine-news/US-Trying-Hard-to-Provide-Proper-Treatment-for-Wounded-Soldiers-22614-1/.

Victoroff, V. M. (1983). *The Suicidal Patient: Recognition, Intervention, Management*. Oradell, NJ: Medical Economics Books.

Waitley, D. (1988). *Seeds of Greatness*. New York: Pocket Books.

Warren, R. (2002). *The Purpose-drive Life: What on Earth Am I Here For?* Grand Rapids, MI: Zondervan.

WebMD. (2009). "Bipolar Disorder Health Center." Downloaded from http://www.webmd.com/bipolar-disorder/mental-health-bipolar-disorder.

Wilkerson, David. (1982). *Have You Felt Like Giving Up Lately?* Grand Rapids, MI: Revell Books.

WJACTV. (2006). Link found between former Soldiers, Motorcycle Deaths." Downloaded from http://www.wjactv.com/news/10325324/detail.html.

Yuan, Nicole P., Koss, Mary P., & Stone, Mirto. (March 2006). "The Psychological Consequences of Sexual Trauma." *National Online Resource Center on Violence Against Women*. Downloaded from http://new.vawnet.org/category/Main_Doc.php?docid=349.